INFECTIOUS DISEASES

MANAGEMENT OF COMMON DISEASES IN FAMILY PRACTICE

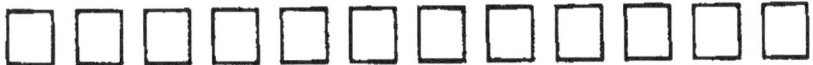

Series Editors: J. Fry and M. Lancaster-Smith

INFECTIOUS DISEASES

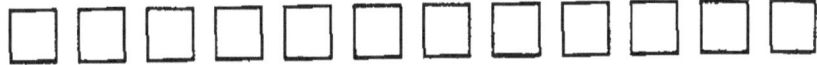

D. Brooks, MD, FRCGP

General Practitioner, Middleton, Manchester

and

E. M. Dunbar, BSc, MB, BS, MRCS, MRCP

*Consultant Physician, Regional Infectious Diseases Unit,
Monsall Hospital, Manchester*

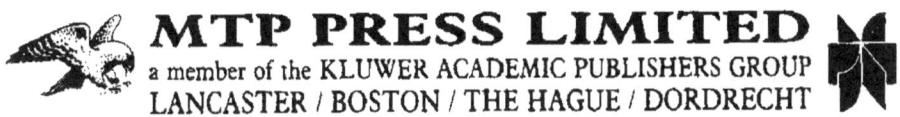

MTP PRESS LIMITED
a member of the KLUWER ACADEMIC PUBLISHERS GROUP
LANCASTER / BOSTON / THE HAGUE / DORDRECHT

Published in the UK and Europe by
MTP Press Limited
Falcon House
Lancaster, England

British Library Cataloguing in Publication Data

Brooks, David
  Infectious diseases. — (Management of
  common diseases in family practice)
  1. Communicable diseases
  I. Title   II. Dunbar, E. M.   III. Series
  616.9   RC111

Published in the USA by
MTP Press
A division of Kluwer Boston Inc
190 Old Derby Street
Hingham, MA 02043, USA

Library of Congress Cataloging in Publication Data

Brooks, David.
  Infectious diseases.

  (Management of common diseases in family practice)
  Includes bibliographies and index.
  1. Communicable diseases.   I. Dunbar, E. M. (Edward
Milne), 1947- . II. Title.   III. Series. [DNLM:
1. Communicable Diseases.   WC 100 B8727i]
RC111.B7 1985   616.9   86-2973
ISBN-13: 978-94-010-8333-1   e-ISBN-13: 978-94-009-4133-5
DOI: 10.1007/978-94-009-4133-5

Typeset and printed by Butler & Tanner Ltd, Frome and London

Contents

□ □ □ □ □ □ □ □ □ □ □ □

Contents

Series Editors' Foreword

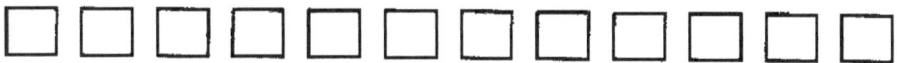

Effective management logically follows accurate diagnosis. Such logic often is difficult to apply in practice. Absolute diagnostic accuracy may not be possible, particularly in the field of primary care, when management has to be on analysis of symptoms and on knowledge of the individual patient and family.

This series follows that on *Problems in Practice* which was concerned more with diagnosis in the widest sense and this series deals more definitively with general care and specific treatment of symptoms and diseases.

Good management must include knowledge of the nature, course and outcome of the conditions, as well as prominent clinical features and assessment and investigations, but the emphasis is on what to do best for the patient.

Family medical practitioners have particular difficulties and advantages in their work. Because they often work in professional isolation in the community and deal with relatively small numbers of near-normal patients their experience with the more serious and more rare conditions is restricted. They find it difficult to remain up-to-date with medical advances and even more difficult to decide on the suitability and application of new and relatively untried methods compared with those that are 'old' and well proven.

Their advantages are that because of long-term continuous care for their patients they have come to know them and their families well and are able to become familiar with the more common and less serious diseases of their communities.

The series aims to correct these disadvantages by providing practical information and advice on the less common, potentially serious conditions, but at the same time to take note of the special features of general medical practice.

To achieve these objectives, the *titles* are intentionally those of accepted body systems and population groups.

The *experience bases* are those of the district general hospital and family practice. It is here that the day-to-day problems arise.

The *advice and presentation* are practical and have come from many years of conjoint experience of family and hospital practice.

The *series* is intended for family practitioners - the young and the less than young. All should benefit and profit from comparing the views of the authors with their own. Many will coincide, some will be accepted as new, useful and worthy of application and others may not be accepted, but nevertheless will stimulate thought and enquiry.

Since medical care in the community and in hospitals involves teamwork, this series also should be of relevance to nurses and others involved in personal and family care.

JOHN FRY
M. LANCASTER-SMITH

Acknowledgements

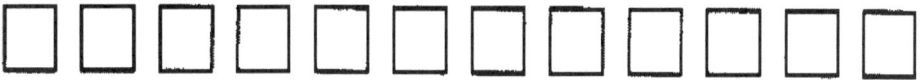

The authors wish to acknowledge their gratitude to Susan Young, editor of the Communicable Diseases Report, for permission to use data previously published there.

Consultant colleagues at Monsall Hospital have been a source of much information and support. Dr Duncan McGee, Consultant Microbiologist at Bury District General Hospital, provided invaluable help with the interpretation of laboratory investigations and Dr Michael Painter, Community Physician, Manchester, provided assistance with our chapter on immunization.

We wish to record our thanks to partners and medical and non-medical staff at the Peterloo Medical Centre for permission to publish practice data.

Finally our thanks are due to our typists Mrs Sheila Marsh, Mrs Helen Bailey and Mrs Lynn Coyne.

DB, ED; Feb. 1986

1

Making a Diagnosis in General Practice

WHAT INFECTIONS DO WE ACTUALLY SEE?

At the Peterloo Medical Centre three principals and two trainee general practitioners provide care for a total of 7800 patients. The age/sex and social class structure are presented in Tables 1.1 and

Table 1.1   Age/sex distribution of practice population

Age (years)	Percentage	No.
Under 5	5.72	446
5 to 14	15.61	1218
15 to 44	40.03	3122
45 to 64	23.43	1828
65 +	15.21	1186

Table 1.2   Social class structure of practice population (percentages)

	Social class					
	I	II	III	IV	V	Never worked
Practice	4	13	53	19	10	1
Great Britain	4	15	53	19	7	2

1.2 and when they are studied it can be seen that the practice structure reflects that of the United Kingdom as a whole with little or no bias.

During 1982, 4574 patients presented with first episodes of infection out of a total of 11 302 first episodes of illness. As a percentage this works out at 40.5. Between one-third and one-half of all new episodes of illness are due to infection, which gives some indication of the prevalence of infection in the community.

Table 1.3 resents these infective episodes classified under the international coding for diseases of the respiratory system, the commonest system involved in infection at 22% of all new episodes of illness. Although it is possible to diagnose some episodes as definite diseases, such as nasopharyngitis or pneumonia, very many episodes must remain at the symptom diagnosis level, e.g.

Table 1.3   Disease of the respiratory system during 1982

	No. of patients	New episodes of illness (%)
URTI	536	4.7
Acute nasopharyngitis (non-febrile)	399	3.3
Acute nasopharyngitis (febrile)	32	0.3
Acute pharyngitis – acute tonsillitis	387	3.4
Acute sinusitis	63	0.5
Acute laryngitis and acute tracheitis	92	0.8
Epidemic influenza	98	0.9
Pneumonia	10	0.1
Pleurisy	6	0.1
Acute bronchitis and bronchiolitis	235	2.1
Chronic bronchitis	15	0.1
Chronic sinusitis	6	0.1
Cough	618	5.5
Sputum – infected	9	0.1
Hoarseness	7	0.1
Total	2513	22.1

cough, because further elaboration is either not possible or not necessary at the time of presentation (see Chapter 4).

Table 1.4 presents the next commonest category, infective and parasitic diseases, at 5% of all new episodes of illness. Fungal infections are prominent in this group but the number of patients with conditions such as mumps, measles and glandular fever will depend on whether there has been an acute epidemic. Surprisingly,

Table 1.4   Infective and parasitic diseases during 1982

	No. of patients	New episodes of illness (%)
Tuberculosis of respiratory system	2	0.02
Gonococcal infections and other venereal disease	4	0.04
Intestinal infective disease, enteritis, dysentery – food poisoning, etc.	47	0.42
Streptococcal sore throat and scarlet fever	4	0.04
Erysipelas	1	0.01
Whooping cough	30	0.26
Measles	35	0.31
Rubella	11	0.10
Chickenpox	40	0.36
Herpes zoster	40	0.35
Mumps	8	0.07
Infective hepatitis	2	0.02
Infectious mononucleosis	1	0.01
Dermatophytosis	88	0.78
Scabies	23	0.20
Viral warts	62	0.55
Intestinal helminthiasis (except enterobiasis)	20	0.18
Other as yet undefined infections	35	0.31
Other recognized infectious diseases not included above	142	1.26
Pyrexia with rash	12	0.11
Pyrexia without rash	44	0.40
Total	651	5.88

four patients presented to us with sexually transmitted disease rather than to a special clinic. Streptococcal throats, infective hepatitis and glandular fever were surprisingly uncommon in 1982.

Table 1.5 presents the category diseases of the nervous system

Table 1.5   Disease of nervous system and sense organs during 1982

	No. of patients	New episodes of illness (%)
Conjuctivitis and ophthalmia	210	1.86
Blepharitis	32	0.28
Hordeolum	32	0.28
Inflammation of lacrimal glands and ducts	4	0.04
Keratitis with or without corneal ulcer	1	0.01
Otitis externa	64	0.57
Acute otitis media	187	1.66
Chronic otitis media	10	0.09
Total	540	4.79

Table 1.6   Diseases of the alimentary tract during 1982

	No. of patients	New episodes of illness (%)
Jaundice	2	0.02
Acute diarrhoea and vomiting	415	3.67
Total	417	3.69

and sense organs – 4% of all new episodes. Otitis media and acute conjunctivitis dominate this section.

Table 1.6 presents data on infections of the alimentary tract. Acute episodes of gastroenteritis predominate in this section. Relatively few patients presented with infective hepatitis.

Infection of the skin is presented in Table 1.7. Boils and carbuncles and impetigo predominate; 2% of all new episodes of illness fall into this category.

Table 1.7   Diseases of the skin and subcutaneous tissue during 1982

	No. of patients	New episodes of illness (%)
Boil and carbuncle	76	0.67
Cellulitis of finger and toe	47	0.42
Other cellulitis - abscess	32	0.28
Acute lymphadenitis	35	0.31
Impetigo	45	0.40
Total	235	2.08

Table 1.8 presents infection within the genitourinary system which accounts for 1.93% of all new episodes of illness. Urinary tract infection is prominent.

Table 1.9 presents only one patient who had a pyrexial illness after childbirth.

Table 1.8   Diseases of genitourinary system during 1982

	No. of patients	New episodes of illness (%)
Pyelitis, pyelonephritis- pyelocystitis	8	0.07
Cystitis, acute	123	1.08
Orchitis - epididymitis	2	0.02
Salpingitis and oophoritis	3	0.03
Vaginal discharge, non-venereal	82	0.73
Total	218	1.93

Table 1.9   Pyrexia of childbirth and puerperium during 1982

	No. of patients	New episodes of illness (%)
	1	0.01

THE DIAGNOSTIC APPROACH

Respiratory infections, infectious fevers, skin infection and urinary tract infection predominate in the community and therefore are reflected in the workload of the general practitioner. Most of these episodes will be diagnosed and managed by the general practitioner without elaborate diagnostic aids and usually without laboratory help. It must also be pointed out that a significant number of conditions such as streptococcal throats, glandular fever and infective hepatitis may well remain undiagnosed due to the presentation of early prodromal symptoms rather than classical symptoms. Nevertheless there would still be no justification for investigating everyone, because management would hardly be affected by the outcome of the tests.

USING THE LABORATORY

In recent years there have been several well-written articles directed at general practitioners on how to use laboratory services. Among the best is that of Ian Farrell (1981), as the central theme of most articles is communication and correct specimen collection.

Most hospital laboratories will provide general practitioners with their own forms and containers, and in the case of bacterial swabs, virology swabs or suspected *Chlamydia* infections will provide the correct transport medium in which to transport the swabs to the laboratory.

In any busy doctor's life, large numbers of forms have to be completed. Hospital doctors in particular are very poor at completing forms correctly, and in competition family practitioners actually usually do a little better. Nevertheless, they are still far from perfect. Most sections are there for a reason and a few extra seconds (it very rarely takes more than a minute) are always worthwhile.

Essential information is names (more than one), type of specimen and date taken, treatment (antibiotics especially) and name and address where the report is to be sent. This is the absolute minimum. Age, sex, length of treatment, previous problems, onset of illness (often essential to the interpretation), intended future treatment, will all aid in a better service. The commonest mistake in hospital practice (EMD) is that the information which appears on the form is different from the information on the specimen (which is often totally unlabelled). It might have been the only specimen the general practitioner sent that day, but when it arrives

Table 1.10 **Infectious diseases units where there is more than one clinical infectious disease physician available**

St George's Hospital Blackshaw Road London SW17 0QT (Tel. 01–672–1255)	St Ann's Hospital St Ann's Road Tottenham London N15 3TH (Tel. 01–800–0121)
Coppetts Wood Muswell Hill London N10 1JN (Tel. 01–883–9792)	East Birmingham Hospital Bordesley Green East Birmingham B9 5ST (Tel. 021–772–4311)
Ninewells Hospital Dundee DD1 1SY (Tel. 0382–60111)	City Hospital Green Bank Drive Edinburgh EH10 5SB (Tel. 031–447–1001)
Ruc Hill Hospital Glasgow G20 9NB (Tel. 041–946–7120)	Seacroft Hospital York Road Leeds LS14 61H (Tel. 0532–648 164)
Fazakerley Hospital Lower Lane Liverpool L9 7AL (Tel. 051–525–2323; 051–525– 5980 – outside normal hours)	Monsall Hospital Monsall Road Manchester MC10 8WR (Tel. 061–205–2393)
	Northwick Park Hospital Watford Road Harrow HA1 3UJ (Tel. 01–864–5311)

in the laboratory it will usually be one in several hundred or even several thousand.

Every general practitioner should be able to discuss his patient with a doctor associated with a laboratory to which the investigations are sent. In most district general hospitals there are now at least two doctors from the pathology specialties. A virologist is the rarest, and the two commonest are histopathologist and haematologist.

Clinical specialists in infectious disease, i.e. a physician with an interest whose special knowledge and experience should encompass all the pathology disciplines when the test is related to the diagnosis or management of infection, are unfortunately rare in the United Kingdom. There are approximately 30, and most are associated with large regional units or, more rarely, university departments (Table 1.10). In the United States this type of physician (tertiary referral physician) is far more common, but in the United States the vast majority of laboratories are run by scientists. On the continent the situation is usually somewhere between the two extremes of the United Kingdom and the United States of America.

In addition to the National Health Service hospitals throughout Great Britain, the Public Health Laboratory system (Tables 1.11 and 1.12) is a very useful and knowledgeable source of information and service to general practitioners. In many parts of the country advice sought on which test for what patient, and how to interpret the result, is best obtained from the closest Public Health Laboratory. Public Health Laboratories usually specialize in bacteriology and virology but are also the usual source of the more rare vaccines and immunizations. It would, of course, be very

Table 1.11   Names and addresses of special laboratories

PHLS Communicable Disease Surveillance Centre (Division of Epidemiology) 61 Colindale Avenue London NW9 5EQ (Tel. 01–200–6868)	PHLS Malaria Reference Laboratory London School of Hygiene and Tropical Medicine Keppel Street London WC1E 7HT (Tel. 01–636–7921 and 01–6363–8636)

Table 1.12   Names and addresses of regional Public Health Laboratories

East Birmingham Hospital
Bordesley Green East
Birmingham
B9 5ST
(Tel. 021–772–4311, ext. 4080)

Level 6
Addenbrooke's Hospital
Hills Road
Cambridge CB2 2QW
(Tel. 0223-242111)

Bridle Path
York Road
Leeds
LS15 7TR
(Tel. 0532-645011)

Withington Hospital
Manchester
M20 8LR
(Tel. 061–445–2416)

Level 6/7
John Radcliffe Hospital
Headington
Oxford
OX3 9DU
(Tel. 0865-60631)

Northern General Hospital
Herries Road
Sheffield
S5 7AU
(Tel. 0742-387749)

Myrtle Road
Kingsdown
Bristol
BS2 8EL
(Tel. 0272-291326; 0272-215411
outside normal hours.) Also
Gonococcus Reference Unit.

University Hospital of Wales
Heath Park
Cardiff
CF4 4XW
(Tel. 0222-755944, ext. 2047)
Also Mycobacterium Reference
Unit.

Fazakerley Hospital
Lower Lane
Liverpool
L9 7AL
(Tel. 051–525–2323; 051–525–
5980 outside normal hours.)

Institute of Pathology
General Hospital
Westgate Road
Newcastle upon Tyne
NE4 6BE
(Tel. 091–272–8811, ext. 297)

St Mary's General Hospital
East Wing
Milton Road
Portsmouth
PO3 6AQ
(Tel. 0705-822331)

Table 1.12—*cont.*

Area laboratories are in:

Ashford (Kent)	Middlesbrough
Bath	Newcastle
Brighton	Norwich
Carlisle	Nottingham
Carmarthen	Peterborough
Central Middlesex	Plymouth
Chelmsford	Poole
Chester	Preston
Coventry	Reading
Dorchester	Rhyl
Dulwich	Salisbury
Epsom	Shrewsbury
Exeter	Southampton
Gloucester	Stoke-on-Trent
Guilford	Swansea
Hereford	Taunton
Hull	Tooting
Ipswich	Truro
Leicester	Watford
Lincoln	Whipps Cross
Luton	Wolverhampton

---

useful for any general practitioner to be able to ring one unit when an infective problem arises, but even when there is a regional unit close enough for regular communication the Public Health Laboratory and a doctor-led laboratory (bacteriology, virology or haematology), are usually on different sites and have different telephone numbers; therefore local choices should be made, built up with local experience of the services available.

Bacteriology swabs

Wound, throat, skin, etc: whenever possible a sample of pus is preferred to a swab. If a swab is taken from a dry infection, moisten the swab with a sterile saline first.

Throat swabs

These are useful only to identify group A beta-haemolytic strepto-coccus, etc. Occasionally, viruses can be isolated, e.g. Coxsackie, echo, mumps, rubella, measles (nasopharyngeal aspirate is better than a throat swab). Even in a hospital environment, when delay should be minimal, the use of a transport medium such as Stuart's for throat swabs for bacterial examination is advisable. Virus transport medium and *Chlamydia* transport medium should be stored in a refrigerator (domestic fridge at approximately 4°C).

Mouth swabs

Mouth swabs are only useful for candida (yeasts) or Vincent's organisms.

Serology tests

A simple clotted blood specimen in a dry screw-top container is sufficient for most investigations. It is particularly important to record the historical nature, i.e. onset of the illness, and when a diagnosis is made on a serological test, i.e. the presence of anti-body or four-fold rise in antibody, two specimens are necessary.

It is an unfortunate fact, but very appropriate, to label the second specimen (usually at least one week, preferably two weeks later) 'convalescent'. This means, of course, that for any acute diagnosis which needs serological confirmation the results are very little use in the management of the patient as the patient should already be recovered. However, to be proven correct carries its own satisfaction and even if proven wrong it may help in the management of future cases. For example negative mycoplasma titres may indicate that the atypical pneumonia treated with ery-thromycin was an ordinary viral pneumonia. Any laboratory in these circumstances should do the other atypical pneumonia titres such as psittacosis, Q fever or even Legionnaire's disease, all of which may respond very well to erythromycin.

If a serological test for acute phase antibodies, i.e. IgM, is available, it can be particularly helpful. The two most noticeable cases are those involving

(1) a recent suspected rubella, particularly in early pregnancy; and

(2) the case of toxoplasmosis where titres may be very high from a *past* infection, even many years ago, and a negative IgM will indicate that it is not the cause of the lymphadenopathy under investigation (see Chapter 11).

Per-nasal swabs (for *Bordetella pertussis*)

Per-nasal swabs are unpleasant for the patient and usually result in a typical paroxysmal coughing spasm. The result of culturing the swab on a chocolate agar plate is often negative but if, in obtaining the specimen, a nasty paroxysm resulted, the patient probably has whooping cough, despite the negative swab.

Even in hospital when transport delays are minimal, only 20% will be positive. A survey in the Regional Infectious Diseases Unit 1977–78, in which EMD was involved, revealed that approximately 40% were positive. However, this result was only obtained by doing three consecutive daily per-nasal swabs and plating the swabs immediately they had been taken (i.e. on the ward). We cannot recommend the routine use of per-nasal swabs in suspected whooping cough in general practice.

Faeces specimens

Faeces specimens are usually obtained with a screw-top container in which a wooden or plastic spoon device, rather like that which used to be used for eating ice cream, is inserted (either as part of the lid or separately loose inside).

The easiest way to obtain faeces for bacterial culture is of course to notify the patient as having suspected food poisoning, and leave the problem to the Environmental Health Officer. This lazy short-cut cannot be condoned for routine use.

'Hot' faecal specimens for parasitology are only really justified when looking for amoebic dysentery and should really be done on site (i.e. actually in hospital – see Chapter 13). *Giardia lamblia* and the more recently discovered cryptosporidia can be found by asking for microscopy of faecal specimens, but this is usually reserved for cases of potential worm infestations when the eggs or ova can be seen when appropriate techniques are used. Again, it would be prudent to warn the laboratory about the particular specimens and what you are actually looking for.

Virology specimens

Virology specimens are very rarely taken in general practice except for rubella serology (see above), and for epidemiological research.

Enteroviruses are best proven with faecal culture and they remain the main differential diagnosis of rubella, which can of course be isolated from a viral throat swab.

Apart from serology, which usually needs two samples at least 10–14 days apart, viral investigation is usually *not* justified in general practice.

Haematological investigations

A simple total white blood count and differential count can be a most useful aid in diagnosing an infection. In general, a neutrophil leucocytosis (total white cell count 12 000 or more with 80% or more neutrophils) would indicate a bacterial infection and a low total count would be in favour of a viral infection. A high eosinophil count (total number greater than 600) would indicate an invasive parasitic disease. (NB: most atopic subjects would have a high eosinophil count.) These are of course generalizations and many viral infections, when seen very early, would have a stress response of a neutrophil leucocytosis. The most notable exception is probably salmonella bacterial infections (including typhoid) which usually produce a low total white blood count, although neutrophils predominate.

Non-specific investigations such as ESR or plasma viscosity can indicate that a patient is ill, and can even be used for following progress, but give no indication as to the nature of the illness.

Specific investigations

Probably the most often used is the screening test for glandular fever (Monospot) but remember (see Chapter 11) that it can be negative for the first 2 weeks of the illness. The presence of atypical lymphocytes on the differential will, of course, be supporting evidence.

Malaria parasites must be specifically asked for, and the laboratories are best warned of the specimen's arrival (see Chapter 13) as the staining and handling of the specimen would usually be different from an ordinary blood count.

Interpretation of results

The interpretation of results will depend on the information given, but the best person to come to a conclusion would be the doctor who ordered the test in the first place. The more information you are able to give your pathological colleagues, the more help they will be able to give you. As always, communication is of the utmost importance.

Always remember, however, that if the history (including contact and exposure) and examination lead the doctor to a conclusion, but the laboratory investigation does not agree with the conclusion, then it is the test or tests which are usually wrong. The tests are often wrong, however, because the specimens have been poorly taken or were the wrong tests in the first place.

Tests for sexually transmitted diseases

Covert sexually transmitted disease is rare in general practice (see Chapter 7) but the following investigations may be helpful:

(1) Microbiological – for gonorrhoea. Take urethral and rectal swabs (not usually done in general practice).

(2) Serological.

Tests are variations on the Wasserman reaction – VDRL and TPHA. The laboratory will usually give some interpretation on past or present infections.

Remember yaws as a possible diagnosis, particularly if the patient has origins in the West Indies or Africa – look for signs of old leg ulcers.

The process of laboratory usage is developed in some detail within the area of urinary tract infection, perhaps the commonest investigation for microbiological assessment in general practice.

The laboratory diagnosis of urinary tract infection

A recent survey of different clinicians dealing with all age groups suggests that only a third of general practitioners who were regular laboratory users send urine specimens from more than 80% of patients in whom they suspect urinary infection compared with nearly all consultants. Those who were selective gave reasons (Table 1.13) and defended their action by saying that patients whom they treated get better, and that bacteriology would not modify the result. It is relevant that 94% of consultants would usually start antimicrobial treatment before the urine report was received, and only 2% of consultants said they would never do this. If a negative report was received after starting treatment, most general practitioners, and about half the consultants, would continue the treatment, either because of a feeling that a course once started should be completed, or because the report was disbe-

Table 1.13 **Reasons for selection given by general practitioners who submitted urine specimens from between 10 and 80% of those in whom they diagnosed urinary tract infections.**

Reasons	No. of general practitioners	Percentage
Patients with recurrent infection	67	99
Diagnostic uncertainty	60	88
Existence of predisposing factor	43	63
Pregnancy	39	57
Age	38	56
Severity of symptoms	34	50
Other reasons	33	49

From Meers, P.D. (ed.), Bacteriological examination of urine. In: *Report of a Workshop on Needs and Methods*. London: HMSO, 1978.

lieved. A bacteriological test of urine after treatment was 'usually' requested by 53% of general practitioners and 82% of consultants.[1]

These observations suggest an important question. Does the selection and screening process that operates before patients reach hospital alter aetiology, diagnosis, management and prognosis there, and so alter the need for bacteriological assessment? (see Chapter 5).

In attempting to answer this question, consideration needs to be given to the question 'what is a diagnosis?' How wide should it be (in physical, psychological and social terms) and how deep should it be in terms of detail required within each category? We also need to consider the aetiology and pathogenesis of ascending urinary infection. The organisms that cause urinary infection are those prevalent in the bowel flora such as *Escherichia coli*, *Proteus*, *Klebsiella and Streptococcus faecalis* (see Chapter 5). Attempts to identify viruses have usually been unsuccessful, but recent work has suggested that organisms with fastidious cultural requirements may occasionally be responsible for some cases of 'abacterial cystitis'.

All patients have common urinary pathogens in the bowel flora, but all patients do not develop urinary infection. The normal urinary tract is resistant to ascending infection which is believed to be the normal mode. Urinary infection is believed to involve the breakdown of defence mechanisms against ascending infection. These include normal voiding, the diluting effect of ureteric urine, and organic acids produced by the mucosal cells of the bladder.

The development of infection within the urinary tract is at present speculative. It is probably a continuous process involving the interplay of potential pathogens, urinary tract defence mechanisms in bladder and urethra, and precipitating factors which interfere with these defence mechanisms - for example, sexual intercourse in women with dysuria and frequency. In a few women symptoms might always be produced solely by precipitating factors. In a few more, precipitating factors might occasionally, or frequently, break down urethral defence mechanisms and a bacterial urethritis might ensue, bacteria infecting para-urethral glands. A large group might alternate between bacterial urethritis and bladder urine infection (which occurs when organisms enter the bladder urine and multiply there) depending on the magnitude of the precipitating factors and the state of the natural defence mechanisms. In another group, bladder urine infection might always tend to develop.

A 'diagnosis' might be made at any stage. Any end-point in this process must be arbitrary (as must any decision about antibacterial therapy).

The concept of significant bacteriuria (the Kass criterion, 10^8cfu/l) tells us that bacteria are multiplying in bladder urine which is a necessary pre-requisite for the development of acute pyelonephritis. This information may not always be necessary or even helpful in management and prognosis. The need for urine bacteriology will vary then according to the type of problem encountered and the type of information needed for management and prognosis, which may differ therefore in women, men and children (see Chapter 5). Women with infrequent attacks of the dysuria and frequency syndrome may or may not have significant bacteriuria, but they are not at risk for renal scarring and kidney failure. Nor is their problem a particularly troublesome one. Why bother to determine the presence or absence of significant bacteriuria either before or after treatment? Therapeutic intervention is hardly a serious matter, especially in view of the trend towards shorter courses, and symptomatic evidence of recovery is all that is necessary. Women with frequent attacks or severe constitutional symptoms should have their urines examined bacteriologically in order to determine the pattern of attacks over a period of time. Are cultures always negative or are some attacks accompanied by significant bacteriuria? Such women can be given a supply of dip slides which can be dropped in at the surgery before commencing treatment.

Since the organisms responsible for urinary infection are those prevalent in the bowel flora, they can be present in the perineum, from where they can acccidentally contaminate the urine during micturition. Since the careful experimental work of Kass in the 1950s, there has been a quantitative basis for the bacteriological diagnosis of urine depending on evidence that bacteria introduced by contamination of a specimen of urine passed per urethra can be distinguished from those multiplying in bladder urine on a numerical basis. The resulting concept of significant bacteriuria (10^8 cfu/l) is now well established in clinical use, but it should be interpreted with caution in general practice for a number of reasons. Different species of bacteria multiply at different rates, and urine is not always a good medium for bacterial growth. Kass was working with a selected population of female hospital patients and he demanded a repeat specimen before accepting any result as significant. Kass's work was not done on women with the dysuria and frequency syndrome, and frequency of micturition can interfere with the validity of the criterion. Bacteria may be involved in a urethral lesion in women (urinary tract infection) and may not get an opportunity to multiply in bladder urine. Finally, bacteria may multiply in prostatic fluid in men, and counts may be low because of the presence of prostatic antibacterial factor (PAF). For these reasons low-count specimens cannot be presumed due to contamination, especially if they are persistent and if they fall in the range between 10^7 and 10^8 cfu/l.

It is the experience of the authors that heavy contamination of a specimen is easily avoided without prior cleansing in most adults in general practice when there is to be immediate inoculation of a dip slide. Nevertheless, the recommended procedure for obtaining a clean-catch specimen involves the following procedures.

Men should wash and dry the glans penis, the prepuce being retracted if necessary. Antiseptics should not be used. The midstream portion of urine is collected or sampled. Females should separate the labia, and the interlabial area should be washed and dried. Antiseptics should not be used. The midstream portion of urine is collected or sampled.

Problems with contamination when they arise tend to occur with the very young or the very old. It is generally accepted that the bacterial count in a specimen of urine changes with time, and since multiplication is a distinct possibility, delay between collection of a specimen and its examination in a laboratory is best avoided. This problem is especially relevant in general practice. As a solution to this difficulty, bacteriostasis by refrigeration at 4°C is clumsy and difficult to apply. The addition of boric acid to urine, producing a final concentration of 1.8%, has also been tried and is commonly used, but it has the defect that a decline in the count can occur, especially after 24 hours when the count can be misleading. It has the advantage that a complete report, including chemical and cytological information and a direct sensitivity test result, can be issued 24 hours after receipt of a specimen in the laboratory. The dip inoculation technique is ideal for general practice and slides can be inoculated by the patient at home (Figure 1.1). The dip slide has the particular advantage that given a suit-

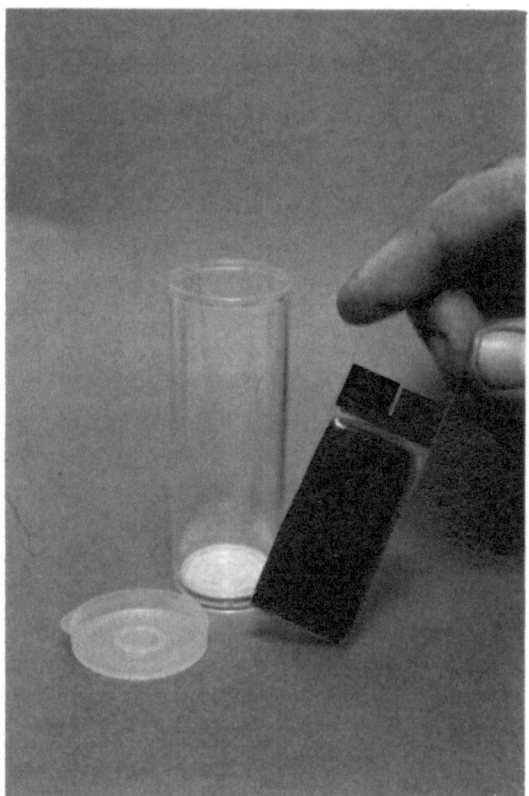

Figure 1.1 A Uricult dip slide

able incubator it can be processed on the practice premises and since the transport problem can be forgotten, there is no disincentive to arrange bacteriological investigation (Figure 1.2 and 1.3). Most clinicians accept that urinary infection must be defined on

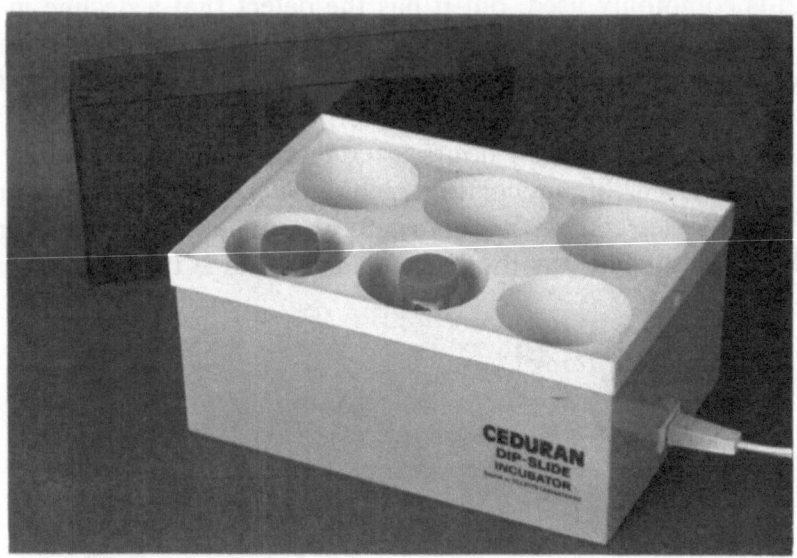

Figure 1.2 A Tillott's incubator

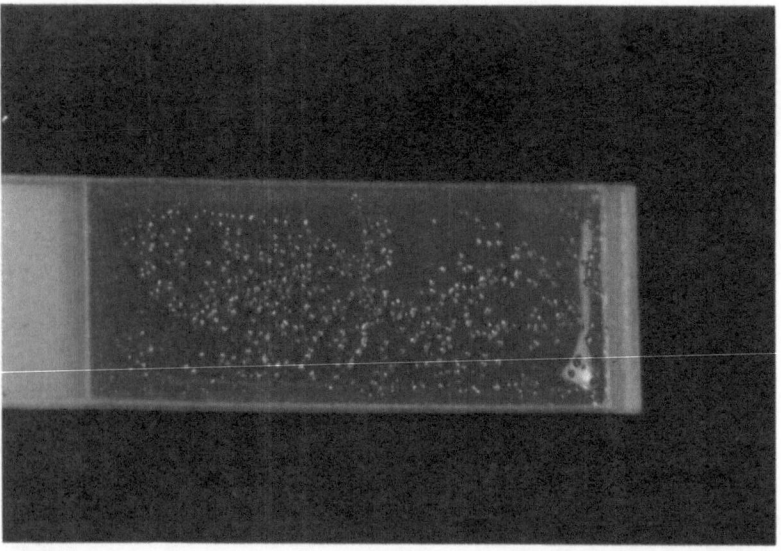

Figure 1.3 An Oxoid dip slide illustrating significant bacteriuria ($> 10^8$ organisms per litre)

the basis of significant bacteriuria. It should be noted that the absence of white cells in a midstream specimen does not exclude bacteriuria.

REFERENCE

1. Farrell, I (1981). Developments and trends in microbiology. *Medicine International*, 387

2

Immunization

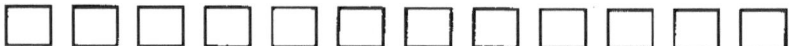

Social change accounts for most of the dramatic improvement during the twentieth century in the mortality and morbidity of the common infectious diseases. However, immunization has played its part and the dramatic fall in the level of protection in the under-5-year-olds after the over-publicized scares of the early 1970s has already led to a major recurrence of whooping cough. It is a great relief that poliomyelitis has not followed.

The balance of the incredibly rare complications versus the vast benefits of immunization should never again be tilted by television journalism, however well meaning. A rational and well-balanced policy towards increasing the immunization rate in preschool children should result in over 90% being effectively immunized.

The immune system has to be capable of an adequate response and 3 months old is the earliest that the basic immunizations should start. BCG is a notable exception.

F.P.C. PAYMENT FEES

Immunization attracts payments in two ways. You can purchase and administer the immunization yourself (as for analgesia). A prescription can be written for the immunization in the same way as for injected analgesia. The prescription is then forwarded to the prescription pricing bureau.

The immunization itself can also attract a fee (as for most of the other vaccinations, except influenza). In the areas where computerized recall operates, a computerized list of patients is sent to the doctor on form V5. Paediatric immunizations for non-computerized children should be detailed on form V3.

The schedule of payments is listed in section 27 of The Statement of Fees and Allowances, where the full procedure is explained. In 1985, the first two triple immunizations attract £2.20 each and the third £3.20. Polio immunization has the same fees i.e. £2.20 each for the first two and £3.20 for the third. The single immunization such as Rubella carries a fee of £3.20, and £3.20 is the standard fee for a 'booster' immunization.

In the case of foreign travel to certain areas, for a patient receiving two typhoid injections the fee would be £2.20 each, and for the patient receiving a single 'booster' injection, the fee payable would be £3.20. International Certificates of vaccination against cholera attract a private fee.

PERTUSSIS

Where the epidemic situation is common, as it is in the United Kingdom in the 1980s, a basic schedule at 3, $4\frac{1}{2}$ and $6\frac{1}{2}$ months is worthwhile. A better and longer-lasting response might be obtained if the schedule were delayed to 6, $7\frac{1}{2}$ and 9–10 months, but it is only worth the delay when a high level of protection and a low incidence exist. Unfortunately, it will be several years before this situation arises in Britain. Booster doses of tetanus and diphtheria should be given at 12–18 months if the earlier schedule is used. It could be given at the same time as the measles immunization for administrative convenience.

For the sake of administrative convenience each district in the United Kingdom is actually considered a high risk or a low risk district and this determines the basic immunization policy. However, children are high risk or low risk, and there may be a high risk child in a district which is considered a low risk district and there will be many low risk children in a district which is considered a high risk district. This is one of the penalties to be paid for having basic immunization schedules under the umbrella of the Community Physicians, whereas the general practitioner would be able to decide on an individual basis whether the child was high risk or low risk.

IMPROVEMENTS

General practitioners should encourage immunization as much as possible, particularly in their less-well-off and overcrowded families. It is an unfortunate fact that those who most need immunization are the last to come forward. Education of support personnel, particularly health visitors, to encourage immunization and active support to gather those who fail to attend will improve most practices' figures.

Computer cards are all very well, but when the computer fails to send for a child for his/her measles immunization because it 'thinks' that only two triples were administered, it is the system that is at fault.

IMPROVING UPTAKE OF IMMUNIZATION

There are positive ways in which the uptake of mmunization could be improved.

(1) Start talking about immunization at the antenatal visits

(2) Mention it again at the 10-day visit postnatally

(3) Try and attempt a firm decision at the 6 weeks postnatal visit

(4) Inform, educate and encourage other members of the health care team to be positive about immunizations

GOVERNMENT ADVICE

Every general practitioner (or at least the practice) should have available the DHSS circular, 31 March 1977, headed 'Precautions to be observed before carrying out immunization procedures', included in the memorandum 'Immunization against infectious disease'.

It is particularly important that any premises on which immunizations take place should have the facilities to cope with an anaphylactic reaction. In the 1980s, 1:1000 adrenaline is hardly sufficient. Intravenous hydrocortisone, chlorpheniramine (10 mg i.v.) and intravenous fluids plus standard resuscitation equipment (Brooks airway, oxygen cylinder etc) should be readily available, as well as the recommended 1:1000 adrenaline. Most people who have an unpleasant experience following an immunization present a very short-lived problem and in adults the episode is often a vasovagal reasponse to having an injection *per se*. However, should a genuine anaphylactic reaction occur, the patient should be given intravenous chlorpheniramine, intravenous hydrocortisone, and 1:1000 adrenaline subcutaneously, as standard. There may be marked bronchospasm and one of the great difficulties would be blockage of the airway through bronchial oedema. A widespread erythematous rash and severe hypotension could result; in these circumstances intravenous fluids may be necessary while urgent transfer to hospital is arranged. Allergic reaction is an incredibly rare situation and is, of course, much more likely to occur in busy hospital departments, e.g. radiology with an unpleasant response to one of the radio-opaque iodine preparations. The general practitioner is more likely to meet this situation if he/she is brave enough to undertake desensitization of hay fever sufferers.

CURRENT ILLNESS

Immunization should be postponed until recovery from any acute illness (particularly if it is a febrile one) is complete. A common cold or 'snuffles' should *not* be regarded as contraindications in this situation. Most children in their first winter of life will have a 'runny nose' for most of the winter. This is all too often the reason why the prime immunizations have not been given, the theoretical reason being that if they have an intercurrent viral infection particularly the poliomyelitis immunization will not work. Since this is theoretical its practical relevance is uncertain.

EPILEPTIC/FEBRILE CONVULSIONS

Epilepsy in the child or first-degree relative is a contraindication to pertussis immunization. Tetanus, diphtheria, polio and measles immunization should be actively encouraged.

Febrile convulsions are also no bar to measles immunization. Antipyretic medication for 3–4 days after the dose may be indicated but there is no justification for reducing the dose, although in exceptional circumstances specific antimeasles gammaglobulin should be administered (concurrently) if there is a definite neurological problem where serious side-effects could be expected.

Epilepsy in relatives should not always be taken at face value. The worst case of whooping cough admitted to hospital under one of us (EMD) in the winter of 1982 was a 9-month-old patient who had not been immunized because an uncle had had epilepsy. Uncle's epilepsy had started at the age of 24 when he had been very fortunate to survive a bad motor cycle accident. The contraindications in the circular issued by DHSS, 31 March 1977, were amended in 1981 to read 'Idiopathic Epilepsy'.

PREMATURITY

A delay in starting immunization schedules in the premature child until the immune system is mature enough to cope is obviously judicious. However, 'delays' should be modified and 2 months is probably the longest necessary unless the child is one of the growing number of neonatal successes less than 30 weeks gestation. A large proportion of these children would not receive pertussis because of 'cerebral problems'.

ATOPY

Atopy, however severe the asthma or eczema may be, is no longer a direct contraindication to any immunization. In the days of antismallpox immunization it was particularly important *never* to vaccinate an atopic individual. Hopefully cases of smallpox will remain as rare as dinosaur bites.

Atopic children should follow the basic schedule. If they are genuinely allergic to penicillin (incredibly rare), the polio immunization may have to be replaced with the deep subcutaneous or intramuscular injections of killed vaccine.

26

Allergy to eggs is a contraindication to measles vaccine, influenza, mumps (very rarely used) and yellow fever.

In practice, particularly with the measles vaccine, egg allergy is hardly ever found to be definite enough to be a contraindication. A 1983 paper in the *Journal of Pediatrics*[1] highlighted that it can be serious; the present authors, however, would not recommend the desensitization procedure be followed, as measles vaccine is not compulsory in the United Kingdom.

LIVE VACCINE

Live vaccines should not be given to any patient who is pregnant because of the risk to the fetus, but very occasionally the risk of exposure to such things as polio or yellow fever may be greater than the risk to the fetus. In these circumstances, the immunization is best left to the specialist referral centre. Live vaccines should never be given to anyone receiving corticosteroids or immunosuppressive treatment (including radiation). They should never be given to patients suffering from malignant disease, particularly those like Hodgkin's (or other lymphomas), leukaemia or other malignancies of the reticuloendothelial system.

Patients receiving inhaled corticosteroids or local steroid ointments can be exceptions.

SYNOPSIS OF VACCINES AND IMMUNIZATIONS

There follows a brief synopsis of each vaccine or immunization available. Remember

ALWAYS check product information
ALWAYS check expiry date and
ALWAYS check for contraindications (to that particular immunization)

Diphtheria

This is a toxoid and as such belongs to the most effective and safe vaccine category. Three doses in childhood and one preschool booster usually confers long-lasting immunity. Diphtheria immunization should not be given over 10 years of age without a Shick test, including a control. Shick negative people who do not require immunization would probably react badly.

Since 1984 a Swiss diphtheria vaccine is now available for adults (UK PL 1511/0915), for which prior Shick testing is not necessary. It is intended for boosting immunity, particularly for medical or nursing staff or paramedical personnel at special risk (a recent diagnosed case.) It contains only a very small quantity of diphtheria toxoid but sufficient to recall immunity. It is available in batches of 10 0.5 ml ampoules, costing, at the time of writing, approximately £2.50 each. The ampoules have a shelf life of about 3 years at domestic refrigerator temperature.

Diphtheria antitoxin immunization is a specialist hospital procedure confined to clinical cases only and is administered with great caution, if at all.

Tetanus

Tetanus toxoid is very safe and very effective. It is generally recommended as a three-injection primary course with a preschool booster. Thereafter every 5 years (when indicated) will probably ensure lifelong immunity. Too many injections will lead to hypersensitivity reactions and these are now becoming more common as the zealousness of Accident and Emergency Departments continues. Even in an accident-prone farm worker who plays football on a field fertilized by horse manure, immunization every three years is still adequate. The difficulty arises for the general practitioner when presented with a penetrating injury (like the ubiquitous rusty nail) when previous immunization is uncertain. When there is even reasonable doubt that previous immunization may be nil, Humotet or antitetanus immunoglobulin should be given, followed by a primary course and accompanied by antibiotic treatment - penicillin by injection at the time. Remember that antibiotics do not kill the spores and it is the germination of *Clostridium tetani* spores some days after the injury that leads to toxin production and clinical tetanus. The spores germinate in anaerobic conditions of secondary infection (*Staphylococcus aureus* using all the oxygen) or a retained foreign body. (Most often both these conditions exist.) There is no substitute for good wound toilet and a strong antiseptic, iodine for preference. It is unfortunate that the only section of the population generally no longer protected are the elderly female gardeners. Equally unfortunately, incredibly rare as tetanus is, the wounds are seldom brought to the attention of any medical practitioner before complications set in.

Measles

This is a live attenuated strain made from virus grown in chicken embryos. It is recommended to be given to children in the second year of life (approximately 15 months). Measles before 9 months is rare due to maternal transplacental gammaglobulin. Egg allergy is a definite contraindication. In children with a history of a *non-febrile* convulsion, immunoglobulin should be given. (Specific antimeasles immunoglobulin should be available from the local Public Health Laboratory.) Children with depressed immunity should not be given vaccine and on exposure should be given specific immunoglobulin (within 3 days).

Some children have a mild measles-like illness but complications with the vaccine are between 12 and 20 times less common than with the natural infection.

Subacute sclerosing panencephalitis appears to have a rate of 0.5–1.0 per million doses of vaccine compared with 5–10 cases per million of actual infection.

If a child is thought to have had measles before the age of 1 year it is still best to give immunization, as – even if the infection was genuine – immunity is unlikely to be lifelong. Adult measles may well become a problem in the near future. Before measles immunization became available, approximately 400 000–500 000 cases were notified annually (this was very close to the actual birth rate). Now there are 200 000 or less and immunization levels, at best, are running at 30–40% in most areas. This leaves a distinct population growing up still at risk.

An effective immunization scheme with 80–90% + uptake would virtually eliminate measles from the UK in much the same way as it has almost disappeared from the USA, where, in 1982, there

29

were fewer than 2 000 cases – 10% of the British cases with four times the population. Of the US cases, 66% were either directly or indirectly related to an imported case from Europe, mostly from the UK.

BCG

BCG is still generally recommended for 11–13-year-olds who are Heaf test negative. Some District Health Authorities are discontinuing the practice of BCG immunization altogether as the incidence of tuberculosis has declined. However, there are certain large sections of the population still susceptible. BCG is recommended *after* birth in many areas to certain ethnic groups, particularly from the Indian subcontinent and refugees from south-east Asia. Although it may not protect completely against the contracting of tuberculosis there is good evidence that it protects the infant against the worst complications of miliary spread and tuberculous meningitis.

In certain circumstances the infant in contact with a very infectious case (usually one or other parent) can be given isoniazid prophylaxis and isoniazid resistant BCG. The giving of BCG is determined by local circumstances and is only done by specially trained and experienced personnel (chest clinics etc). The general practitioner rarely meets a BCG problem except after immunization when the injection has been either (1) too deep, or (2) too superficial.

(1) Too deep can lead to a BCG abscess with collection of pus as a hard lump or some discharge. The practice of giving BCG in the right arm should alert the general practitioner to this possibility if the child appears to be using the left arm, as reluctance to use the limb may actually be the only symptom. (Perhaps BCG should be given in the left arm to left-handed families.) The practice of using the right arm stems from the use of the left for other immunizations (the now defunct smallpox etc).

Oral isoniazid, for 1 week as a single daily dose of 10 mg/kg, will help solve the problem.

(2) Too superficial injection can lead to a persistent ulcer. The

manufacturers recommend local iodine treatment (Betadine paint), but sometimes this is insufficient and *local* isoniazid powder applied directly will clear it up. Isoniazid powder is usually available from local hospitals where it will be used for making isoniazid syrup and comes in 20 g sachets. A single sachet would be sufficient when applied over the 3 or 4 necessary days.

Rubella immunization

Rubella is a *live* attenuated vaccine and is first offered between the ages of 10 and 14 (see above, for contraindications to live vaccines). The vaccine is offered to girls *only* in the UK not only on economic grounds but also because, theoretically, continued exposure whilst protected will boost immunity – males being the source of continued exposure.

A history of rubella *without* virological isolation or serological proof is as much use as a chocolate teapot. At least a dozen other viruses (mostly ECHOs and Coxsackies) can give exactly the same picture as classical rubella (see Chapter 11).

The vaccine comes in two versions – (1) almevax (RA 27/3 strain) which appears to be a better producer of antibodies but has a slightly higher rate of side-effects (rubella-like illness) than (2) cendevax. Almevax is probably the best for routine childhood immunizations and cendevax is mostly used for selected groups of adult females (postpartum antibody negative). Rubella immunization should never be given to any patient who might be pregnant and pregnancy should be avoided for 2 months afterwards. However, there is no recorded case of congenital rubella following immunization.

Family practitioners could increase their uptake of rubella immunization not only by using age-sex registers to offer it to all their 10-year-old girls – they should also logically offer it to all adult females with their second prescription of oral contraceptives (not the first, because oral contraception is not effective for the first month).

Influenza immunization

The DHSS recommendations for influenza vaccine are wide-ranging and the number of patients who could be immunized in any one practice in their recommendations is quite large. The authors, however, recommend that the General Practitioner concentrates on his patients with chronic lung disease and any patient, e.g. a steroid dependent asthmatic, who would probably need hospital admission should they suffer a bout of influenza. Chronic lung disease should include those patients with chronic 'wet' lungs, e.g. patients with congestive cardiac failure. It would be worth noting on a patient's medical card and placing them upon the list for influenza vaccine if they have a hospital admission for a chest condition. The DHSS recommendations for patients with chronic lung disease and diabetes would need modification on an individual patient basis and in the case of chronic renal disease advice from their specialist physician would be necessary.

Influenza vaccine is an inactivated surface antigen vaccine. It usually contains three strains and at least one is usually varied every year dependent upon the WHO recommendations and likelihood of the dominant strain that particular winter. General Practitioners receive no FPC fees for administration of influenza vaccine but they can make a small profit by acquiring a number of doses and receiving a prescribing fee. It is most important not to use last year's vaccine. The best time to administer the vaccine is late autumn, i.e. late October/early November.

Other immunizations

In addition to hepatitis B immunization (see Chapter 9) and rabies immunization (see Chapter 13) there are a few other less usual immunizations which general practitioners may be asked about.

(1) Anthrax in slaughter house, glue factory or dock workers. It is a relatively ineffective killed bacterial vaccine and not generally recommended even if obtainable

(2) Leptospirosis vaccine is sometimes sought by sewer workers – again a killed bacterial vaccine and relatively ineffective (many stereotypes)

(3)   Meningococcal vaccine is sometimes suggested during out-
      breaks but most meningococcal infections in Britain are type
      B (see Chapter 10), and only A or C immunizations are
      available. A combined A and C immunization may be avail-
      able in the UK in the near future but its use may well be
      strictly limited (possibly for health care workers going to
      developing countries, like the Sudan, with a known seasonal
      problem)

General practitioners should only normally do the routine immunizations (see Table 2.1) and specialist advice should be sought and
ought to be readily available for any other problems.

Table 2.1   Example of immunization schedule for use in UK

Age	*Vaccine*	*Comments*
During first year of life	Dip/tet/pert and oral polio vaccine	Need three doses of each of these. Start immunization at 3 months old. Give second dose at 4 months & final dose at 6 months. Interval is not absolute: providing child receives three doses at some stage before first birthday immunity will be effective. However, this should be regarded as the extreme rather than the norm. NOTE ANY CONTRA-INDICATIONS
Second year of life	Measles	Not less than 4 weeks after another live vaccine
School entry/ entry to nursery school	Dip/tet booster Oral polio booster	Preferable to give at least 3 years after basic course
Between 11 & 13	BCG	Many authorities no longer do this routinely. There is case for it in areas of high risk or following discovery of TB case in a school
Between 10 & 14	Rubella	Girls only Allergy to rabbit and neomycin (–cendevax)

Table 2.1—*cont.*

Age	Vaccine	Comments
		Allergy to neomycin and polymyxin (–almevax)
On leaving school	Oral polio vaccine Tetanus	Booster Do not give if recipient has received a dose within last year. If full basic course has not been given by this age then arrange for it to be done. Following a full basic course immunity may be lifelong but boosters are given at intervals of 5–10 years. Reactions may occur in the overimmunized
Child bearing	Rubella	Women only. Screen with serological testing first, as 90% will be immune. **BE CAREFUL ABOUT IMMUNIZING WOMEN WHO MAY BE PREGNANT**
Adulthood	Immunization for foreign travel	See relevant chapter
Adulthood	Influenza vaccine	See text N.B. No F.P.C. payment

REFERENCE

1. Herman, J. J., Radin, R. and Schneiderman, R. (1983). Allergic reactions to measles immunization in patients hyperective to egg protein. *J. Pediatr.*, **102**, 196–199

3

Self-care

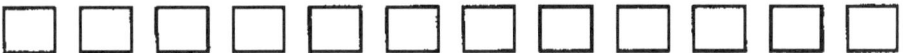

WHAT IS HEALTH?

Over the past couple of decades, two different views of health care
have been adopted by the theorists. The first, and perhaps the
commonest, held by medical and non-medical people alike, is to
equate health with the absence of sickness and therefore to see it
as a product of medical care. There is a powerful infrastructure
bolstering this concept. First, undergraduate medical education
extols the virtues of technological medicine at the expense of community care, in terms of curricular time and influence. Second, we
are concerned largely with the hospitals as centres of care and
spend 70% of our NHS budget developing them. Third, powerful
commercial interests, such as the drug industry and the surgical
instrument industry, tend to preserve the *status quo*. Fourth, media
coverage glamorizes high technology medicine: ratings are higher
for heart transplants than for a routine visit by a health visitor.
Finally, the development of private medicine, which not unnatur-
ally focusses on high revenue surgery, tends to confirm the view
that health is essentially a process of symptom swatting.

Those with wider responsibilities, such as the World Health
Organization, realize however, that health is a product of the
complex interaction between political, economic, social and educational forces. In 1968 WHO defined health as a 'state of complete physical, mental and social well-being' and not merely as the

absence of disease, a state which the symptom-swatters claimed was achieved rarely and then only fleetingly – perhaps during moments of orgasm!

Although it is easy to dismiss the social model as unattainable, it is also obvious that the medical model is almost valueless in the Third World countries where health has far more to do with clean water, sound drains, and decent nutrition than it has to do with doctors. What is less immediately obvious is that the medical model, as Illich pointed out[1], may have decreasing relevance for the developed world despite its obvious successes such as immunization programmes, hip surgery etc.

A shift in emphasis

Burkhart (1983)[2] has pointed out that our health care system needs a change of emphasis from illness to health, from cure to prevention and care, from treatment to health promotion, from episodic treatment to continuous treatment, from specialists to general practitioners, from doctors to nurses and social workers, from specific problems to comprehensive care, from single-handed doctors to primary health care teams, from clinical decision making to community participation, from professional domination to lay care and self-responsibility.

This shift in emphasis is necessary for a number of reasons, not least the increasing difficulty in financing the health service which we already have. Perhaps most important, however, is the need to increase the dignity of the patient as a person and make him less dependent on doctors and professionals for health care so that he comes to realize that health is very largely a product of his own efforts. Curative medicine after all is faced with the problem of the law of diminishing returns. We are paying more and more for less and less. Treatment-orientated research is slowing down. Twenty years ago one pharmaceutical component in 4000 might have been expected to reach the market. Now the figure is one in 12 000. The prospects for prevention and self-care are very good but are rarely tried.

INFECTIONS AND SELF-CARE

What are he strategies that we can employ to promote the concept of self-care with regard to infections? Catling (1982)[3] has given us five.

The need to identify

First we must identify the major health issues, priorities and programmes that are relevant. What are the common infections in the community? (Chapter 1). How can they best be treated? Why do people come to the general practitioner for treatment when the diseases they have can be treated at home? Do doctors prescribe unnecessarily or inappropriately? Who are the people with responsibility for promoting health at primary care level? How can the common infections be prevented?

The need to involve

We must involve everyone, professionals, universities, members of health authorities and community health councils, the media, the public and of course the individual. If the media can change public attitudes negatively about whooping cough vaccine, they can change public attitudes positively towards health promotion. The environment must be a learning atmosphere. Health must be marketed in a professional fashion.

The need for information

We, as professionals, need information about advances in knowledge but so often that is where we stop. The media and the public need information about the state of health care in the UK and they need to know what they can do about it. The Health Education Council and the pharmaceutical companies produce a good number of valuable educational leaflets about many common illnesses and infections. How many copies have we in our waiting rooms? How often do we reinforce our advice with suitable reading material? Do we make sufficient use of the waiting room which should be a learning environment for the patient? So often the walls contain notices which seem to be limited to telling patients not to upset the doctors by doing this, that or the other and not to spit on the floor! Is there anything more useful they could learn? Are we making sufficient use of local newspapers and local radio? The word 'doctor' comes from the Latin 'docere', to teach, and perhaps we should be doing more of it.

The need for investment

We must be prepared to invest in advancing programmes of proven benefit. Currently £8.5 million (less than 0.2% of the NHS budget) is spent through the Health Education Council, the principal avenue of government health promotion, compared with £100 million spent on advertising by the tobacco industry.

There is also a need for investment of time. The 5-minute consultation ought to be a relic of the past. We need help from others in order to reduce workload, realign resources and modify traditional medical education so that new ideas about primary care involving disease prevention, health promotion and self-care can be implemented.

The need for innovation

There is a need for innovation in order to improve the effectiveness of programmes and the commitment of individuals. If we are to reduce prescribing for simple upper respiratory tract infection we need to offer something in the consultation which is seen as more valuable. This will often require the acquisition of new skills and new consultation techniques and new attitudes towards our role in the community. Vocational training and continuing education will need to reflect these ideas.

THE PRACTICE AS A LEARNING ENVIRONMENT

All practices have an atmosphere - good or bad. All practices have a 'shop window' which can be seen from the outside looking in. Stand outside your practice and take a look at it. What is the practice attitude towards home visits? re appointments easy to get when your child is ill? Are surgeries held at convenient times? What is the attitude of receptionists towards patients? - towards each other? How do they get on with the doctors? What are relationships like betweeen the doctors? If I am told to treat my child's cough myself by Dr X on Monday, do I know that Dr Y will give me antibiotics on Tuesday? Is the atmosphere inviting when I walk in? Look at the waiting room walls. Does everything you read seem to be a litany of 'don'ts' or is the waiting room a bright informative place in which to sit? Some practices have browsing boards as well as notice boards. Reading material should relate to health care. Would the local library consider an exhibition of health care titles? What about the use of video material or at least tape/slide demonstrations? Does the practice have a patient participation group? What about lectures from practice team members on common childhood infections and how to manage them at home?

Some helpful material

1. Immunization programmes

All practices should have notices, booklets an handouts, relating to immunization programmes for infants and children and for foreign travel. Many of the sponsored newspapers produce notices relating to immunization for foreign travel which can be displayed in practice premises. All notices of this type should be supplemented by information relating to the way in which the practice organizes its clinics.

2. Common childhood infections

Handout leaflets and notices can be obtained or, better still, prepared by the practice. Drug companies will often be prepared to contribute to the cost of printing. If the practice does not believe that chickenpox or mumps should necessarily be seen by the doctor, patients need advice on how to recognize it and manage it and when the doctor should be involved (see Chapter 11).

3. Coughs and colds

If the practice believes that patients should manage the infection themselves, why not help the patients to learn how to do it? Patients should be made aware that any worries or complications deserve a consultation (see Chapter 4).

4. Gastrointestinal infections

Many patients with these conditions would not attend the surgery or send for a visit if they knew what to do. The practice should do the teaching. Much of that teaching should involve the need for fluid replacement and the avoidance of antibiotics (see Chapter 8).

5. Sexually-transmitted diseases

Leaflets containing appropriate advice (Chapter 7) could be handed to many women asking for oral contraception or presenting with a vaginal discharge and, of course, many men worried about minor blemishes on the penis, as long as the general practitioner had the skill to introduce the topic.

6. Home medicines

Practice information systems could well include recommended home remedies for minor ailments such as coughs and colds, diarrhoea or sore throat.

POSTSCRIPT

The word 'doctor' means 'teacher' and the authors hope that readers will use this book to design practice information systems for their patients which will lead to more self-care. All systems should state briefly what the problem is, how it can be prevented, how it can be treated and when patients should see the doctor.

PATIENT INFORMATION

Morrell, D. (1981). *Minor Illness and How to Treat It at Home.* (London: Health Education Council)
Fry, J. and Fryers, G. (1983). *The Health Care Manual. A Family Guide to Self-care and Home Medicines.* (Lancaster: MTP Press).

REFERENCES

1. Illich, I. (1977). *Limits to Medicine. Medical Nemesis: The Expropriation of Health* (Harmondsworth: Penguin)
2. Burkhart, S. (1983). 'Primary Care: Is it poor care for poor people?' *Br. Med. J.,* **286,** 195-6
3. Catling, J. (1982). *Progress in Health Promotion. United Kingdom and abroad. Report of a Symposium held by the Faculty of Community Medicine of the Royal College of Physicians of the United Kingdom.* Wessex Regional Health Authority

4

Respiratory Tract Infections

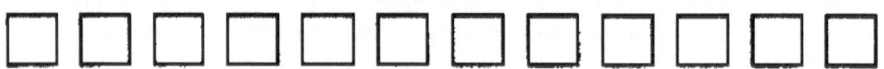

Respiratory infections are common in general practice. In DBs practice 22% of all new episodes of illness and 55% of all new episodes of infection are due to infections of the respiratory tract. For every 1000 patients registered with a general practitioner presenting during the course of any given year, 140 will consult with acute upper respiratory infection, 75 with acute throat infections and 62 with acute chest infections; a further 28 will consult with acute otitis media and in a non-epidemic year five will consult with influenza. For every 1000 patients on a general practitioner's list, 20 will present with an acute chest infection during any given year, eight will be admitted to hospital and one will die.

Respiratory tract infection is therefore a good area for practice audit. What should our standards be? Are we managing our patients according to these standards? Is our prescribing as it should be? Are we admitting the right patients to hospital and in good time?

AN APPROACH TO DIAGNOSIS

A major problem for the trainee general practitioner on entering general practice is that classifications, diagnostic and management behaviour that he has acquired (which may have been suitable for undergraduate education and clinical behaviour with a referred population in hospital) will confuse rather than help patient management in general practice. The general practitioner sees much respiratory illness that is vague and self-limiting and defies easy classification in the way to which he has become accustomed in hospital. Precise anatomical or pathological diagnoses are often impossible and when they are not they are difficult to justify. In general practice, patients are best classified by the way they present (Table 4.1).

Table 4.1 A clinical classification of respiratory infection in general practice

Children
acute upper respiratory infection (cough, colds)
croup
acute throat infections
acute ear infections
acute chest infections

Adults
acute upper respiratory infection (cough, colds)
influenza
acute sinusitis
acute chest infections
chronic chest infection
bronchiectasis
chronic bronchitis

CHILDREN

Acute upper respiratory infection

Acute upper respiratory infection is the commonest reason for children to be brought to see the general practitioner. The commonest symptom is a cough and parents worry because they are afraid that the cough will 'go down on the chest' and because coughing interferes (they believe) with sleeping, which in turn will 'interfere' with growth. Nasal symptoms, such as a blocked or running nose, are also common and are a source of near panic in

43

some mothers with new babies, such mothers may well lie awake all night listening to the snuffles of a newborn baby for fear that they might stop – indicating that the baby has 'choked'. Malaise, headache and fever may be noticed and the latter particularly may give cause for concern to a parent, particularly if there is a history of febrile convulsions.

Assessment

Two basic questions need to be considered. First, what is the parent worried about? It is startling to discover as a result of patient questionnaires just how frequently parents leave a doctor's consulting room without indicating their cause for concern. Simple attempts by the doctor to elicit symptoms are not enough. The second question is, is there anything that the doctor needs to worry about? All children who present with upper respiratory infection require a chest examination, throat examination and otoscopy. Laboratory examination is usually pointless unless undertaken for research purposes. There is little correlation between various symptoms and signs and a variety of viruses such as influenza, parainfluenza, respiratory syncytial virus, coronavirus, Coxsackie A and B, rhinovirus and adenoviruses which have been incriminated in these diseases.

Management

In recent times we have seen increasing patient frustration with medical technology and an increasing realization among doctors that a 'traditional' medical approach is often inadequate in general practice. Nowhere is the need for 'holistic' medicine more apparent than in the management of acute upper respiratory infection in children. The scientist could simply point to the study by Stott (1979).[1] He studied 965 consecutive upper respiratory infections in children aged under 10 years, in detail. Significantly different management plans made by seven doctors did not correlate with clinical outcome as judged by complication rates, recall rates and demand for treatment for similar episodes in the future. Overall about 40% received antibiotics, 30% cough mixtures or decongestants or both, and 30% advice alone. No patient group appeared to benefit by the criteria selected. Doctors who prescribed antibiotics for 20% of upper respiratory infection in children had similar crude complication rates to those who gave antibiotics to 60% of such cases. The proportion of patients returning for further treatment (24% within 6 months was similar for each of the seven doctors' patients, suggesting that the mother's decision to seek help for future episodes of upper respiratory infection was either influenced uniformly by each of the doctors or was not influenced by the doctor at all.

What should the general practitioner do?

Strict adherence to the 'scientific method' might suggest a nihilistic approach, but this is mistaken. Schofield[2] and his colleagues have identified a series of consultation tasks (Table 4.2) which should

Table 4.2 Achieving greater 'breadth' in the consultation: A list of seven consultation tasks

---

1. To define the reason for the patient's attendance in physical, psychological and social terms:
   (a) nature and history of problems
   (b) aetiology
   (c) patient's ideas, concerns and expectations
   (d) effects of problems

2. To consider other problems:
   (a) continuing problems
   (b) at risk factors

3. To choose an appropriate action for each problem

4. To achieve a shared understanding of the problems with the patient

5. To involve the patient in management and to encourage him to accept appropriate responsibility

6. To use time and resources appropriately:
   (a) in the consultation
   (b) long term

7. To establish or maintain a relationship with the patient which helps to achieve the other tasks

---

(Schofield, 1983)[2]

be attempted in all consultations, and their use is well exemplified by the management of upper respiratory infection in children.

Tasks 1 and 2. The first two tasks involve drawing up a problem list for the patient and the family. What are the causes for concern for the patient, the parent and the doctor? As a result of talking with and listening to his patients, whether parent or child, the general practitioner might learn that a 3-year-old girl had started to cough, especially at night, some 3 days earlier. She also had a 'runny nose'. From his records the doctor might learn that the child had a history of recurrent 'wheezing' and that a partner frequently prescribed antibiotics for recurrent 'colds'. Further 'listening' could reveal that mother had a 'weak chest'. i.e. 'recurrent bronchitis', as a child and that she wanted a course of antibiotics 'like Dr X prescribes' to help the cough and to prevent 'bronchitis'. Clinical examination is unhelpful, apart from very mild generalized 'wheezing' only audible on auscultation. The family live in poor-quality terraced housing and father is unemployed.

Tasks 3-7. Tasks 3-7 enable solutions to emerge to identified problems. Clearly a decision whether to prescribe an antibiotic is a relatively small part of the total management of the above scenario in general practice. Usually, however, undergraduate and early postgraduate education have together contrived to make it loom large as the most important decision as far as the doctor is concerned. The doctor is then so preoccupied with his problem (whether to prescribe an antibiotic) that he is unable to identify the patient's problems. It is doubtful that antibiotics would help very much but the management skills required of the doctor are that he should enable the parent to 'see this', and at the same time learn something about the possible role of allergy in the pathogenesis of the symptom. If an antibiotic is prescribed it will be defended on two grounds: first, because of the poor social circumstances and greater risk of a chest infection and, second, because the general practitioner was unable to remove the mother's anxieties about the need for antibiotics in one consultation.

What about cough medicines?

In 1980 the general public in the UK spent £19.3 million on over-the-counter cough medicines. On any given day, 12% of adults and 17% of children are taking over-the-counter cough medicines. In 1981, 13 505 000 scripts were issued by general practitioners for expectorants and cough suppressants at a cost of £14 771 000.

The prescribing of cough suppressants and expectorants is a contentious issue in general practice. Whatever their efficacy (and many children's medicines are placebos), there is no doubt that the prescription teaches the parent that medicines are 'necessary' and the family will tend to consult the doctor again and again for trivial future self-limiting coughs. Proper attention to tasks 5 and 6 is crucial if we are not to produce a population who, to use Illich's phrase, are suffering from 'social iatrogenesis'. In addition, the issuing of a prescription is often a way of avoiding the more time consuming tasks involved in defining the problems and identifying the solutions.

It may well be in the particular case described above a prescription for a cough medicine will be totally ineffective and that a bronchodilator might be more appropriate.

Other measures

Opportunistic health education should concentrate on good ventilation in the bedroom and the avoidance of excessively cold air and variable temperatures. The child should not have to live in rooms filled with tobacco smoke. Good hydration is important and the parents should appreciate the need to give an adequate supply of fluids.

Self-care and prevention should be major management themes but realistic advice about whether and when to consult if symptoms are severe or prolonged should also be given. Popular myths dictate that colds and coughs should disappear in 2–3 days – whereas the parents should be aware that, providing there is no deterioration in the child's condition, there is no need for anxiety: coughs may well take 2–3 weeks to settle.

Croup

Acute inflammatory obstruction of the upper respiratory tract in children is commonly the result of croup. Table 4.3 presents a differential diagnosis.

Table 4.3 A differential diagnosis of upper airways obstruction in children

1. Croup
2. Epiglottitis
3. Large infected prolapsing tonsils
4. Peritonsillar abscess
5. Retropharyngeal abscess
6. Foreign bodies
7. Angioedema glotti

Presentation

All these conditions can present with stridor but the usual mode of presentation for croup is a telephone call from an alarmed parent in the small hours of the morning. Indeed, stridor presenting during the day requires an *immediate* visit as it is probably not croup. The parent will comment on the noisy and difficult breathing and the stridorous child may well be heard in the background.

Viral croup presents in children between 9 months and 3 years and prodromally there may be mild coryzal symptoms and fever. A barking cough is usual, especially at night. Typically, the stridor fluctuates but it tends to be worse during sleep.

Assessment

The usual scenario is that the child will be sitting on mother's knee and the child is best examined initially from a distance and in this position. The first thing to do is to establish the history. Acute epiglottitis is usually of very sudden onset but may be preceded by a sore throat and fever and accompanied by expiratory grunting. *Haemophilus influenzae* is the causative organism. The patient becomes toxic, drools saliva and secretions and prefers to sit forward, as is the case with a peritonsillar abscess or a retropharyngeal abscess.

The next decision is to establish whether the stridor is mild, moderate or severe. Moderate stridor is accompanied by subcostal retraction, a slight tachycardia and rising tachypnoea. Severe stridor may be less noisy (due to exhaustion) but is accompanied by subcostal and suprasternal retraction with use of accessory muscles. The child may be cyanosed. Tachycardia is more than 120 per minute and bounding and the child is very anxious and possibly stuperose.

Management

Any diagnosis other than viral croup (Table 4.3) will almost certainly require hospital admission. All are rare, however, with the exception of viral croup, so that a decision about hospital or home management is commonly necessary. Mild to moderate viral croup can be managed at home along the following lines.

Home management. It is first of all necessary to establish the concerns and expectations of the parents. What do they feel about hospital admission? Are their concerns realistic and can you manage them? Will the parents be able to cope with the effects of the problem, which will almost certainly involve a very disturbed night, and are they intelligent enough to know when to contact you again if necessary? The next task is to ensure that the parents achieve some understanding of the process of the disorder and what is happening. The term 'inflamed larynx' or 'voice box' can be useful.

Given this understanding, the parent can then be actively involved in management. Fluids, preferably hot drinks, are helpful and aspirins can be given, but antibiotics and steroids are of no value. Steam inhalations are traditional and often surprisingly helpful, despite the fact that clinical trials have been unable to establish their value. However, appropriate clinical trials are very difficult to set up. Recent measurements of total respiratory resistance before and after treatment with nebulized water in five children with viral croup showed no improvement.[3]

As subjective improvement is usual and as parental involvement is worth encouraging, steam inhalations using Karvol capsules or a teaspoonful of 'Vick' in a container of boiling water is recommended. The bowl can be held under the child by the mother. Before leaving the home, the general practitioner should ensure that the mother can identify signs of increasing stridor and know how to contact him.

Referral to hospital. If a decision is made to refer a child to hospital because of the nature of the diagnosis or the severity of the stridor, the parent will be fully aware of the reason and should accompany the ambulance. Oxygen may be given orally by mask during the journey and the hospital should be aware of the nature of the emergency.

Pharyngitis and tonsillitis

The term 'sore throat' implies discomfort and difficulty in swallowing food or fluids and, as a result, when severe it may be accompanied by excessive salivation. The severity of the symptoms is related to the virulence of the pathogen (which may be bacterial or viral) and the extent of the pharyngeal and tonsillar involvement. Exudates may be seen on the tonsils in both viral and group A β-haemolytic streptococcal disease.

Antibiotics or not?

When *Streptococcus pyogenes* is considered to be the infecting organism, penicillin (or erythromycin in sensitive patients) is the treatment of choice. Parenteral penicillin should only be considered in the presence of significant toxicity, which usually indicates a peritonsillar abscess.

Unfortunately, there is no way in which we can be certain of the diagnosis, which means that some patients with viral infection will be given penicillin and some with streptococcal infection will not. There are a number of helpful statements which can be made in this situation.

(1) It is probably true that many unnecessary prescriptions for penicillin are given because of the fear of complications of streptococcal upper respiratory infection. This fear should not be a consideration. First, rheumatic fever is extremely rare. Second, a recent general practice study revealed that only 16 cases of nephritic syndrome occurred in 500 000 patients over 3 years. Only four were associated with a recent history of sore throat, and one of the children had been given a full course of penicillin whilst the other three had not been seen by a general practitioner at all. In any case, it is very doubtful whether the acute nephritic syndrome which is associated with β-haemolytic streptococcus infection ever progresses to chronic glomerulonephritis.

(2) In the light of the above statement, the best guides to whether or not an antibiotic should be prescribed are:

(a) the clinical severity of the illness,
(b) the presence of continuing problems or associated risk factors, whether social or physical,
(c) parental expectations.

The toxic and prostrate child should be given penicillin or erythromycin. Less severely ill children may justifiably be given antibiotics if the social circumstances (housing, family size, parental intelligence) are detrimental. Parental expectations may seem an odd indication. In view of the general practitioner's continuing relationship, however, it is pointless to get into a violent quarrel with a parent who cannot see that penicillin is unnecessary. The general practitioner must use his bargaining skills and consultation skills to educate his patients and to identify the real causes for concern. This may need more than one consultation.

(3) Perhaps the most important thing is to ensure that you only prescribe penicillin or erythromycin; never be seduced into prescribing any other antibiotic however glib the excuse.

Since long term complications are unlikely, a five-day course of penicillin is usually adequate in general practice.

Prescriptions for other things

In most situations the main aim of any consultation for these conditions must be to share one's understanding of the condition with the patient and to involve the patient and family in management and to encourage them to accept responsibility. By taking this approach one is conserving health service resources not only in the consultation but also long term.

Aspirins, throat lozenges and linctuses are therefore best not prescribed. In order to maintain a relationship with a patient, however, a prescription may on occasion be necessary, particularly in association with financial hardship (FP 10s are free under the age of 16) but the patient must never be misled into thinking the prescription is necessary for clinical reasons.

Acute ear infections

Acute otitis media is *par excellence* a disease of general practice. In the United Kingdom 99 out of every 100 patients seen are managed solely by the general practitioner. It follows that diagnostic criteria and management norms recommended by hospital doctors and supported only by studies on the one out of every 100 patients seen by them are likely to be quite inappropriate in the community.

Presentation

Figure 4.1 indicates annual consulting rates for acute otitis media in general practice. The incidence rises rapidly with age to reach a peak at about 6 years and declines rapidly thereafter. There is also a seasonal incidence (Figure 4.2). In any practice about 40% of all children will suffer from acute otitis media during their first decade. It is more common in poor and large families.

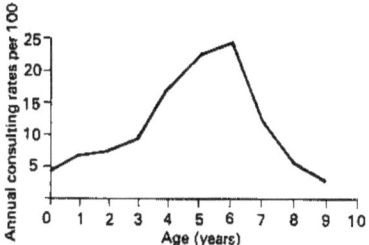

Figure 4.1 Annual consulting rates for acute otitis media

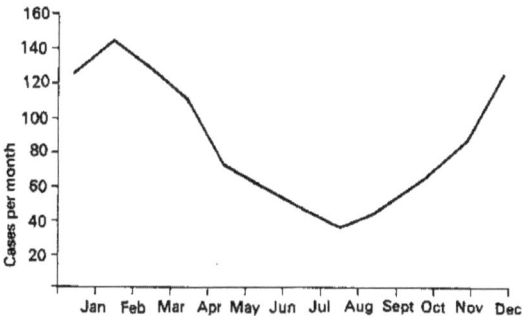

Figure 4.2 Seasonal incidence of otitis media

Assessment

The usual presenting complaints are pain in the ear, deafness, malaise and pyrexia. Inevitably the behaviour of the general practitioner will be influenced by whether the attack is acute or recurrent and by the time of day when symptoms present. All appointment systems should allow a child with earache to be seen promptly. If the drum is seen before perforation it may be very red and bulging. After a perforation there will be pus in a normal external canal and, after cleansing, a perforation may be visible with discharge exuding from it.

Fry describes four clinical types on assessment[4]: 70% of children have earache with an intact red drum, 20% have a discharge, in 5% deafness is a presenting feature, and about 5% (infants) are acutely ill, feverish and generally distressed. In this context, the advantages of using a head light with aural speculae are worth considering. Both hands are free for cleansing the external canal with a Jobson Horne probe and cotton wool and the rare but potentially dangerous attic perforation can be spotted.

It is sound practice to examine both ears and to ask the mother whether she feels that hearing is impaired, and to attempt to assess the degree of deafness by whisper test or tuning fork.

Management

Management is controversial. There is no doubt that the vast majority of children with otitis media, whether viral or bacterial, settle down spontaneously and quickly with little or no residual damage.

It is difficult to find evidence that antibiotics modify the outcome. Indeed, Van Buchem *et al.*, in a double blind study in children published in 1981[5], failed to demonstrate any advantage in prescribing antibiotics. It is hardly surprising therefore that yesterday's arguments about which antibiotic to prescribe, and by what route, were never fully resolved and that today's argument is whether to prescribe antibiotics at all. What is clear is that statements sometimes made by hospital specialists recommending parenteral antibiotic therapy for otitis media do not reflect general practice experience and should not be followed. In 18 years' general practice experience by one of the authors (DB), parenteral therapy has never been necessary for acute otitis media.

The bacteria isolated from cases of acute otitis media are presented in Table 4.4. Organism may vary with age. The authors recommend the following management approach. Pink drums and earache should be managed by appropriate advice about analgesia. Toxic symptoms and bulging red drums should be treated

Table 4.4 Organisms responsible for acute otitis media

Organism	Frequency (%)
Pneumonococci	54
Haemophilus influenzae	32
Group A β-haemolytic streptococci	7
Staphylococcus aureus	1
Others	6

with co-trimoxazole or amoxycillin in short courses of 3-5 days. Chaput de Saintonge and colleagues (1983) demonstrated that a 10-day course of amoxycillin was no more effective than a 3-day course[6].

Out of hours calls

What should the practitioner do when he is awakened at 3.00 a.m. and told that a 6-year-old child has earache? The authors' approach after taking a clear history is to advise adequate analgesics (which will rarely have been given) and to reach agreement with the mother that she will phone back for an immediate visit if the pain does not settle within 30 minutes. The parent should be advised to bring the child to the surgery the following morning. Failure to reach agreement, or a second phone call, are rare. Adequate analgesia means an adult aspirin or paracetamol tablet for a child of this age.

Follow-up

Follow-up consultations after 5-7 days should be aimed at observing normal drum resolution and reassessing deafness. About 17% of general practice episodes are associated with hearing loss. The drum may remain pink and dull and deafness may stay for several weeks. Complications such as mastoiditis, intracranial sepsis and chronic suppuration are very rare. Further investigation or ENT referral are most unlikely to be needed but should be considered in children with more than four attacks each year. Adenoidectomy may be considered.

Secretory otitis media

Secretory otitis media or glue ear is common. About 11% of 2-year-olds have been suspected of having the disorder on otoscopic findings and on the basis of the flat compliance graph of tympanometry. Onset is insidious and the child may present at school with a behaviour problem, slow learning or 'switching off' during lessons. Hearing may fluctuate, so audiometric tests should be easily available in the community and frequently repeated.

Aetiology and pathogenesis are obscure. The middle ear is filled with thick, sticky mucous material causing deafness. Poverty and air pollution appear to be involved and there is a seasonal and geographical variation. Infection, eustachian obstruction and allergy have all been incriminated.

Referral to an ENT surgeon is necessary. The mainstay of treatment has been the insertion of grommets, which are effective in resolving hearing loss, although spontaneous resolution does occur. At the same time, it should be pointed out that the condition can recur and several insertions of grommets may be needed. (In recent months, the use of grommets has been challenged.) Co-trimoxazole (Bactrim; Septrin) is effective and with an antihistamine/decongestant preparation may well be a suitable first line treatment in general practice.

Acute chest infections

The presence of chest signs such as wheezing and crepitations can be confusing. In the United Kingdom acute bronchiolitis occurs in epidemics during the winter. It affects up to 1.5% of infants predominantly between the ages of 1 and 6 months and very rarely beyond 12 months. All cases are due to viruses, with 80% caused by respiratory syncytial virus. The presenting features are cough, wheeze and considerable respiratory distress as evidenced by rib and substernal recession and the use of accessory respiratory muscles. Management is symptomatic and there is no indication for antibiotics. Hospital admission may be needed for respiratory distress.

Bronchitis

Although viruses may replicate in the bronchial mucosa during upper respiratory infection, we now know that when a cough is associated with wheezing the most likely diagnosis is asthma. Therefore the most useful treatment is bronchodilators, and antibiotics are unhelpful.

Acute pneumonia

Virus pneumonia is common and in the vast majority of cases is relatively insidious in onset and associated with little respiratory distress or subsequent mortality or morbidity. Secondary bacterial infection is rare, therefore antibiotics have no place in management. The exception to this statement is in association with an influenzal illness when a severe staphylococcal pneumonia with a high mortality can occur. Adenovirus infection can occasionally cause severe bronchiolitis.

Mycoplasmal pneumonia is common in patients over 5 years. Characteristically the symptoms are mild and the clinical signs pronounced. Serological testing will confirm a diagnosis and the treatment of choice is erythromycin for 2 weeks.

Streptococcal pneumonia is the commonest bacterial pneumonia producing lobar consolidation. The treatment of choice is penicillin. If this is given parenterally, the resolution of signs and symptoms should be very rapid.

H. influenzae type B pneumonia may be lobar or scattered and will respond well to many antibiotics including erythromycin, amoxycillin or co-trimoxazole.

Some guidelines

A surprisingly large number of children with chest signs and mild illness are suffering from a viral bronchiolitis or pneumonia and antibiotics are not needed. In older children, when the illness is mild and the signs marked, a mycoplasmal pneumonia may be suspected and the child treated with erythromycin. A lobar pneumonia is usually streptococcal and responds well to penicillin. Any child who is significantly ill is best managed in hospital where a search can be made for underlying causes, whether host factors or in the environment. It should be noted that the common general practice tendency to give broad spectrum antibiotics to all children with chest signs is difficult to justify.

COUGHS AND COLDS IN ADULTS

When 'hospital doctors' experience their first general practice 'surgeries', a major difficulty many of them face is understanding why so many adults present with self-limiting coughs and colds and sore throats.

Patients tell us that they want to 'catch it in time', 'stop it going onto the chest', 'get a good night's sleep' or simply 'get something stronger in order to stop it'. There are other reasons for attending, however. How is it that the same patient will stoically cope with several acute episodes of upper respiratory infection over a period of many months or even years and then for no apparent reason attend a surgery saying that he wants something to stop it? It must have been these infections that the psychiatrist, Michael Balint, had in mind when he exhorted general practitioners to try to see presenting symptoms, not only in terms of diseases but also in terms of personal conflicts and problems and then use that understanding to produce a therapeutic effect. At a simple level this might mean that the real reason for attendance in a man with a 3-week cough is a fear of cancer or tuberculosis. Moreover, however, the patient has very limited insight into why he or she 'does not feel well'. Perhaps the sore throat is simply the last straw in a whole chain of events which have been bothering the patient and finally precipitated a surgery attendance. Occasionally an important event like a trip abroad or a business meeting or a 'new date' may be threatened by the early symptoms of infection and make effective treatment urgent and imperative.

Management

The inexperienced doctor will see these consultations as a battle with his patients about whether or not an antibiotic is needed or whether or not any prescription is needed. This is a pity, because this approach is self-defeating. No relationship of trust and confidence is ever built up with the patient, a relationship which must be carefully nurtured if the doctor is to be effective in the future.

The present authors would prefer to offer their readers an entirely different challenge. From what has been said already it is clear that these consultations offer enormous scope for health education and self-care and if this is to be done effectively, while maintaining and strengthening a relationship of trust, the need is for the exhibition of considerable interpersonal and consultation skills.

The first task must be to identify the real reason for attendance, to define the problems well enough to draw up a problem list. What are the patient's ideas, concerns and expectations? If your trainee or your partner gave a prescription 8 weeks ago for the identical symptoms, you are going to have an uphill struggle trying to convince the patient that you don't need to prescribe anything. Do make sure that you allow the patient to describe the effects of the symptoms on his/her daily life. What does all this prevent him from doing? What is the thing that bothers him most about the symptoms? How does he consider that you can best help?

There really is no need to put on a 'psychotherapy hat' when dealing with these problems. The patient may well be just 'trying you out' with a simple problem and wondering whether she can tell you about something much more important to her – but pointed and probing questions about how often she has inter-course, and whether she enjoys it, will give you nothing, only a reputation for being 'a bit queer' with your patients and 'a bit of a laugh' with your colleagues. Perhaps the crucial thing is to be open to your patient's ideas so that space can be provided for the patient to work in and discuss whatever she wants to. Remem-ber that despite all the above truths the patients may know no-thing other than the fact that she wants you to get rid of the cold!

The examination

While you have been listening to the patient you will have had ample time to carry out an examination. The examination itself is as comforting to the patient as the opportunity to talk about the problems and should never be neglected. Pulse, throat, sinus ten-derness, ears and chest should all receive careful attention. The patient must always believe that the symptoms are being taken seriously.

Having defined the problems accurately in terms of their effects as well as their pathology, and considered continuing problems and risk factors, the doctor must then share his understanding of the problems with the patient and together they must choose an appropriate action for each problem. The patient must come to understand the natural history of viral upper respiratory tract infection, the limits to the interventions that doctors can make and just how much they can do for themselves.

The prescription

In view of the need to encourage self-reliance and to avoid dependency, not to mention the need to conserve the nation's economic resources, the ideal is to send the patient away without a prescription. To do this, however, both you and the patient must feel that something much more valuable was gained during the consultation and if the challenge you accept is to create this understanding (rather than see the challenge as avoiding a prescription) you stand a fair chance of success. Do not be afraid of giving advice about smoking or hot drinks and aspirins. If the patient seems to want a cough medicine, there is no reason why you should not select a cheap one and ask them to buy it. It may cost them less than an FP 10, which currently costs £2.00!

Occasionally, however, a prescription will be required. Have the sense to realize it when you are failing to reach agreement and do not get into a battle over something like this. You may have saved the country the cost of a cough medicine or even a few penicillin tablets but the patient has not seen it your way, will not consult with you again and could well get them at another consultation with a colleague. You have in fact 'lost' if this happens, whereas if you give the prescription at least you survive to try out your skills with the same patient another day.

Some useful cough medicines

In all fairness it has to be said that the value of cough medicines on or off prescription is unclear. The fact that studies have failed to demonstrate any measurable benefit does not mean that none exists and your medical skill might best be employed in selecting something cheap and harmless from the enormous range available that you can prescribe, or your patients can buy.

The dry and painful cough that accompanies the acute phase of upper respiratory infection may well be eased by linctuses containing syrup, volatile oils and perhaps codeine or some related drug such as pholcodine. 100 ml of simple linctus, 5 ml q.i.d., at present costs 60p and 100 ml of pholcodine linctus, 5 ml q.i.d., costs £1.00. Compound preparations should be avoided. There is no evidence of any superior effect and the only discernible difference between them and the preparations mentioned is more expense and more side-effects.

Mucolytics are no more effective than steam inhalation and, if an expectorant is desired, steam inhalations using hot water and 'Vick' (or Karvol capsules) are best advised. These are particularly helpful in tracheitis.

INFLUENZA

Influenza is a febrile illness which lasts 4–6 days or sometimes longer. There is an incubation period of 1–3 days and it is caused by Type A, B or C influenza virus.

Although sporadic and locally-based infection occurs throughout the year, attacks are mild and indistinguishable from other acute upper respiratory infections. Influenza is important because of the epidemics that occur. Over the past four centuries it is believed that there have been about 30 world pandemics and very many more disrupting epidemics which occur unexpectedly every 4 or 5 years. In the United Kingdom in 1957 an epidemic with a new strain of A2 Hong Kong influenza virus involved 10 million of our then 50 million population and there were 5000 deaths, mostly from secondary bacterial infection in the elderly. The cost then to the nation was £100 million.

Practice management

The treatment and eventual arrival of a new influenza epidemic is a challenge to the practice administration and a nightmare to any general practitioner. There is much that should be done.

1. Patient education

In the great majority of cases influenza is benign and self-limiting and patients must be made aware of this. National and local campaigns in the media should advise the community of the natural history of the condition, suggest self-help measures and indicate when medical help should be sought. Campaigns should ask the public to avoid non-urgent consultations to allow for increased pressure on doctor time.

2. Prevention

Vaccines against A influenza are available and many public organizations and private companies encourage their employees to have annual inoculations. Indeed, with some companies the annual 'jab' is a status symbol akin to a company car, an office carpet or lunch in the executives' dining room and an indication that an employee's efforts are 'valued'. This may well be the only measurable benefit from the vaccine, as the value of the procedure has yet to be established. Official DHSS guidelines are to immunize vulnerable groups such as cardiac and respiratory invalids and the elderly. High risk patients may benefit from amantidine 100 mg. b.d. orally for 1 week when given before the onset of symptoms. Although it prevents the patient feeling ill, it allows infection and antibody formation to occur.

3. Modifying practice workload

Epidemics arrive insidiously, often in late autumn or early winter, and sporadic cases present intermittently and may continue over a period of 6–10 weeks. By the end of the second week house visits and consultations may be up by a factor of three or four; the practice is virtually under seige and may well be short staffed as team members succumb themselves. Normal work and standards are under severe pressure in the community and in hospital; less immediately urgent matters such as 'sick notes', release courses for trainees, outside jobs and screening clinics may on occasion need to be abandoned.

Assessment and management

Outside epidemics, influenza is extremely difficult to separate from other respiratory conditions. Typically, the onset is acute with sudden tiredness, abnormal coldness, aching muscles and a headache. Rhinorrhoea and pharyngitis are relatively uncommon but rigors and heavy sweats are not. Typical symptoms are more usual in the young adult and the middle-aged. There is a range of response starting with mild malaise and culminating with severe prostration, the elderly being particularly vulnerable to complications such as pneumonia or even heart failure and myocardial infarction.

At present, though common and distressing, the infection is benign and has few complications and a low mortality for most people. The condition improves over 4–5 days with fluids, analgesia and rest. Patients seen at home should be examined and advised how to manage themselves and told to contact the surgery if the expected improvement does not occur or if the condition deteriorates. Re-visits are necessary only to those at special risk. The high risk patients should be given flucloxacillin 250 mg q.i.d. for 10 days.

ACUTE SINUSITIS

Infection of the sinuses is overdiagnosed, poorly understood and badly treated in general practice. Much so-called chronic sinusitis is in reality nasal allergy and the term 'recurrent acute sinusitis' is preferable.

Streptococcus pneumoniae and *H. influenzae* are the comonest infecting organisms although anaerobes may be involved. *Streptococcus milleri* is a facultative anaerobe. Presenting features are those of an acute coryza complicated by systemic disturbance of an unusual degree, purulent nasal secretions and facial pain. It is usual to be able to demonstrate tenderness on percussion over the site of the sinuses involved, whether infraorbital or supraorbital. The maxillary sinus is most frequently involved, followed by the ethmoidal frontal and sphenoidal. About 10% of cases of maxillary sinusitis result from dental infection. Diving and swimming in infected water may precipitate an attack, as may barotrauma. Anatomical abnormalities and nasal obstruction or swelling due to allergy may obstruct the draining ostia of the sinuses leading to stagnation and infection.

Diagnosis and management

The history should include an enquiry about facial pain; facial tenderness on percussion over the affected sinus is usual. Purulent material may be seen in the nostrils and the patient will often volunteer that the condition seems more upsetting than the average 'cold'.

Penicillin is the antibiotic of choice and it should be continued for 10–14 days. Nasal drops of 1% ephedrine and oral decongestants such as Sudafed are helpful; moderately potent analgesics may be needed. Continuing discomfort and recurrent attacks require further investigation with sinus radiology and an ENT opinion.

CHEST INFECTIONS

The term 'chest infection' is popular with both doctors and patients. Patients like it because a cold 'on the chest' sounds a much more likely explanation of the way they feel than a simple cold in the nose and a much more respectable reason for going to the doctor. General practitioners like it because 'noises in the chest' on auscultation seem to justify the administration of an antibiotic and provides a clear-cut guideline as to whether they should or should not be prescribed. Several myths need to be destroyed.

The first myth is that auscultatory adventitia in the chest implies chest infection. In many instances cough, expectorate and wheeze may be the manifestation of allergy. This is very frequently the case in children, but even in adults much so-called 'bronchitis' is allergic in origin.

The second myth is that secondary bacterial infection in patients with viral pneumonia is invariable. This does occur in influenza, for example, and in acute exacerbations of chronic bronchitis.

Patients with other chronic respiratory diseases such as bronchiectasis and cystic fibrosis may have permanent bacterial colonization of the respiratory tract and this may be provoked by viral infection. In other situations the concept is open to considerable doubt.

Assessment

Fry (1983) points out that he can distinguish four clinical 'groups' of patients with acute chest infections using Papworth's 'guessing tubes'[4].

(1) The first group of patients with 'acute wheezy chests' have diffuse and bilateral signs, largely 'rhonchi' and occasional interspersed moist sounds which may clear on coughing.

(2) The second group comprises patients with 'local moist sonds' which are inspiratory and may be coarse rales or fine crepitations. These sounds are usually found at one or other lung base but they may occasionally occur in more than one area.

(3) A third group may present with a pleural rub, with consolidation with an effusion or with signs of collapse. These are a small proportion of the total.

(4) The fourth group are the patients with acute chest infection who have no physical signs but have signs of probable chest infection on X-ray, i.e. pneumonia.

It might be added that patients can also be classified according to their presentation. Some may have little systemic disturbance and the chest signs might be a chance finding on auscultation. Others may have significant toxic symptoms and may be lying prostrate in bed at home. Others may have a past history of chest disorders such as bronchiectasis and cystic fibrosis. Other patients may be vulnerable because of their age.

Some recognizable clinical syndromes and their management

Pneumonia

The average family doctor (general practitioner) will see more bronchopneumonia (widespread, patchy changes) than primary lobar pneumonia, although the latter still accounts for the majority of hospital admissions[7].

Most of the patients will be prescribed an antibiotic, particularly those who produce purulent sputum (see Chapter 1), although only normal flora is likely to be found on culture. Asthmatics can, of course, produce 'purulent' sputum which is full of 'eosinophils'. Other patients with chronic chest disease, mainly bronchitics but also bronchietatics, should probably have a semisynthetic penicillin, such as ampicillin or Amoxil, in bigger doses, 500 mg q.d.s., than those used for urinary tract infections, as they hope to penetrate purulent sputum. It must also be remembered that patients with congestive cardiac failure can have crepitations from infection as well as congestion.

As stated above, the staphylococcus is a very important cause of mortality, particularly in influenza epidemics as a secondary invader, and even with measles an antistaphylococcal antibiotic is often added (i.e. ampicillin plus cloxacillin) if the patient is particularly unwell. The signs to look for are tachycardia, as well as tachypnoea and poor peripheral circulation (cold, clammy skin and weak pulse). The patient is often using accessory muscles extensively. Most experienced general practitioners will have no difficulty in recognizing the acutely ill bronchopneumonia sufferer, whether the patient has had a bad chest problem before or not. Almost all these patients will go to hospital and the most difficult decision that a general practitioner has to make in these cases is not whether they need an antibiotic (or which one) or whether they need a chest X-ray, but whether they need hospital admission.

The most important aspect of the treatment of a chest infection is not parenteral antibiotics, nor the ready availability of oxygen and X-rays, but physiotherapy. Good physiotherapy many times a day (usually depending on the patient's strength), concentrating if possible on certain areas dictated by X-ray, is probably the most important single aspect of therapeutics more readily available in hospital than in the patient's home.

Lobar pneumonia

Acute lobar pneumonia caused by the pneumococcus, with a short history, usually only a day or two of pleuritic chest pain, shortness of breath, fever, even rigors, accompanied often, but not always, by physical signs of consolidation, is still *best* treated with intravenous benzylpenicillin. This usually results in dramatic improvement within 24 hours. It is still the commonest cause of primary pneumonia in hospital and still carries an appreciable mortality. It is most often fatal in the very young and the very old. The most significant thing about the mortality in these patients is that those with positive blood cultures have a mortality many times that resulting when the blood cultures are negative. Most of the patients who die are dead before the blood culture results are known, and therefore intravenous benzylpenicillin forms part of the treatment of most severe pneumonias.

Atypical pneumonia

The atypical pneumonias are so called because they do not behave like pneumococcal pneumonia. The physical signs and chest X-ray findings and general well-being of the patient are often at odds. The commonest odd combination is a relatively well patient with a terrible X-ray, but the opposite can be true. The X-ray can show considerable consolidation when there are no signs.

Mycoplasmal pneumonia is the commonest, but psittacosis, Q fever, legionnaires' disease and even adenovirus and influenza can be indistinguishable on X-ray and acute laboratory findings (white count, electrolytes etc). The only real clue can come from epidemiological evidence, particularly a known outbreak – legionnaires' disease from a certain hotel, psittacosis in someone exposed to birds (not only the psittacine variety), Q fever with abbatoir and other animal-associated occupations.

It must be remembered that two thirds of legionnaires' disease cases in the United Kingdom are native to this country, but a lot of these are in association with a known outbreak. The average general practitioner is more likely to see a case in somebody who has recently been away from home, particularly a hotel holiday.

Many other clues quoted are irrelevant. EMD has seen herpes simplex complicating all the above pneumonias, not just pneumococcal.

Treatment. Erythromycin is the treatment of choice initially, particularly in children, but adults can have tetracycline, unless legionnaires' is suspected. If the patient is ill enough to consider the use of rifampicin, which is probably the best all-round antibiotic for atypical pneumonia, he or she needs to be in hospital.

If psittacosis is generally suspected (the clinical clue could be splenomegaly) then the patient should be admitted to isolation facilities, as person-to-person infection is very well documented.

Acute on chronic bronchitis

The responsible organisms are *H influenzae* and pneumococci. Ampicillin is the drug of choice in a dose of 500 mg q.i.d. for 7 days.

Further management. Chest 'radiography' may help to confirm a diagnosis, localize the lesion, assess progress and to exclude other conditions such as cancer or tuberculosis. Only about 10–20% of patients are admitted to hospital; therefore, if the patients respond to treatment investigation may be delayed until the convalescent period. Physiotherapy is important. If there is no improvement after 24 hours, hospital admission will be necessary.

It should be noted that chest signs may take a month to clear, despite the patient feeling almost completely recovered. It is not necessary to continue antibiotics until the chest signs have gone. Indeed, antibiotics may cause a continuing fever. Concurrent treatment may be necessary for heart failure or associated bronchial spasm.

All patients should be followed up either at home or at the surgery until chest signs have disappeared.

REASONS FOR CHEST X-RAY

Initial X-ray

Initial X-ray is indicated occasionally if the diagnosis is in doubt, particularly if atypical pneumonia is suspected, but most importantly if there is any reason to suspect carcinoma (smoker, weight loss, clubbing) or tuberculosis (contact history, weight loss).

Clearance X-ray

A clearance X-ray is particularly indicated if the patient has taken longer than 10 days to get better. This should also include children, particularly those who have had measles which needed an antibiotic (a small minority).

Whooping cough is probably the most difficult as it lasts 2–3 months regularly (particularly the nocturnal cough). If the child is not gaining weight and able to behave normally, particularly in the daytime, a chest X-ray is indicated long before the end of the illness and occasionally may have to be repeated.

An abnormal chest X-ray may lead to hospital admission for investigation (e.g. bronchoscopy) but most often should lead to a course of antibiotics and physiotherapy.

REFERENCES

1. Stott, N. C. H. (1979). Management and outcome of winter upper respiratory tract infections in children 0-9. *Br. Med. J.* 1, 29
2. Schofield, T. (1983). The application of the study of communication skills to training in general practice. In *Doctor Patient Communication.* Pendleton, D., and Hasler, J. (eds.) p. 259 (London: Academic Press)
3. Lenney, W. and Milner, A. D. (1978). Recurrent wheezing in the preschool child. *Arch. Dis. Child.* **58,** 468
4. Fry, J. (1985). *Common Diseases. Their Nature, Incidence and Care.* 4th Edn (Lancaster: MTP Press)
5. Van Buchem, F. L., Donk, J. A. M. and Vant Hoff, M. A. (1981). Therapy of acute otitis media. Myringotomy antibiotics or neither. A double blind study in children. *Lancet,* **2,** 883-7
6. Chaput de Saintonge, D. M., Levine, D. F., Temple Savage, I., Burgess, G. W. S., Sharp, J., Mayhew, S. R., Sadler, M. G., Moody, R., Griffiths, R., Griffiths, S. and Meadows, G. (1982). Trial of three day and ten day courses of amoxycillin in otitis media. *Br.Med.J.,* **284,** 1078 ·
7. Macfarlane, J. J., Finch, R. G., Ward, M. J. and Macrae, A. D. (1982). Hospital study of adult community-acquired pneumonia. *Lancet,* **3,** 255

5

Urinary Tract Infection

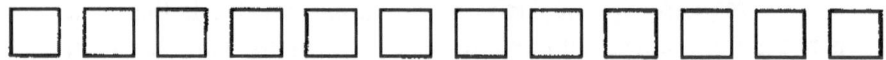

INTRODUCTION

Urinary tract infection is experienced and studied at three different
levels and is commonly encountered at all of them. First of all
there is the community itself; a survey carried out in Wales in
1969[1] revealed that nearly half of a screened population of 3000
women between 20 and 64 years had experienced dysuria (defined
as a burning pain on micturition) at some time in their life. Twenty
per cent had actually complained of dysuria during the year
preceding the study and in half of them the symptoms had lasted
2 weeks or more. Self-medication was very common and *only 10%
of the women with symptoms in the year of the study bothered to
consult a doctor.* These figures were confirmed in a more recent
general practice based study published in 1983 involving 6000
women between 20 and 54[2]. On a 62% response, 20% reported
dysuria in the year preceding the study and half of them suffered
at least one further episode in the same year.

The second level is the experience of the general practitioner.
When urine is examined bacteriologically using the Kass Criterion
of significant bacteriuria, the total incidence of symptomatic infection is 12.5 per 1000 patients at risk per year. Table 5.1 presents
the incidence of urinary infection symptoms and urinary infection

Table 5.1 Incidence of urinary infection symptoms and urinary infection by the Kass Criterion in women, men and children in the author's practice

Patient	Symptoms per 1000 patients at risk per year	Infection per 1000 patients at risk per year
Women 15+	48	25
Men	10	4
Girls	40.2	7.7
Boys	17	3.8

in the author's (DB) practice in women, men and children. The incidence in women peaks in the 15–25 age range. The incidence in men rises with age.

The final level is the level of specialist referral. Table 5.2 demonstrates that less than 10% of patients with urinary tract infection are referred to hospital specialists. However, paediatricians, gynaecologists, physicians, urological surgeons and geriatricians will all have views on the management of these common infections which relate to their own experience of them.

Table 5.2 Referrals from general practice of patients with cystitis and pyelonephritis, per cent

Clinical diagnosis	Action taken by general practitioner		
	Admission to hospital	Outpatient referral or domiciliary visit	Laboratory investigation
Cystitis	0.5	3.4	43.4
Pyelonephritis	1.7	6.3	55.6

From RCGP OPCS (1974). *Morbidity Statistics from General Practice 1970–1* (London: HMSO)

SOME CONSEQUENCES OF THESE LEVELS OF EXPERIENCE: AN OVERVIEW

Our understanding of the nature, course and outcome of any disease process will obviously depend upon the study in patients of the development of symptoms and signs over a period of time. This process, when linked with a record of changes in appropriate scientific measurements, whether biochemical, histopathological or immunological, will define the aetiology and pathogenesis of the basic disease process even further, and knowledge so gained can then be used to produce diagnostic criteria and management norms which can be recommended and supported for use in clinical practice. However, as already mentioned, medical care is divided into a primary care and a secondary or hospital care system and this has inevitably had a significant influence on this process; knowledge and clinical standards gained by a study of one population cannot necessarily be applied to the other unless bias introduced by population selection can be excluded with certainty. This concept applies with particular relevance to urinary tract infection which, as we have seen, is primarily a community problem. In the past, firm statements about the prognosis of this disease process have been made supported only by studies on hospital patients and error has been introduced. For example, we now know that there is no evidence that recurrent attacks of dysuria and frequency in women lead to kidney failure. Although general practitioners did not find evidence to support this assumption[3], hospital experience led us to believe otherwise[4].

Even the aetiology of urinary infection can vary between hospital and general practice as a result of the referral process, as Table 5.3 illustrates. If they are to be relevant, diagnostic criteria and management norms for general practice must be based on experience with general practice patients. For example, when managing women with the dysuria and frequency syndrome in general practice, an approach recently offered by a hospital specialist[5], comprising a careful history, physical examination (including a pelvic examination), a bacteriological diagnosis and a high vaginal swab to exclude gonorrhoea, may be less helpful in managing general practice problems than it would be in managing hospital ones, relating as they do to women with very frequent or atypical symptoms who had been referred for a second opinion.

If we are to derive diagnostic criteria and management norms and set standards for care in general practice, we cannot do this without considering the role of the general practitioner in the

Table 5.3 **Urinary pathogens in general practice and in hospital practice during 1977**

General practice % age of total infections	Organisms	Hospital practice % age of total infections
73.1	*Escherichia coli*	40.9
6.0	*Staphylococcus albus*	6.5
5.7	*Proteus mirabilis*	10.8
4.8	Klebsiella	13.6
3.4	*Streptococcus faecalis*	12.1
3.0	*Enterobacter/Citro-*	
	bacter spp.	3.9
1.4	Pseudomonas	4.8
0.9	Streptococci	
	(non-faecal)	2.2
0.7	*Proteus vulgaris*	2.0
0.4	*Staphylococcus aureus*	
	(coagulase positive)	2.5
0.4	Others	0.6

Based on 2110 hospital and 435 general practice infection episodes. Figures supplied by courtesy of Dr S. J. Eykyn, Dept. of Clinical Microbiology, St Thomas's Hospital, London, SE1 7EB

community (Table 5.4). Society requires direct and easy access to a low cost non-hierarchical system of care provided by a primary health care team with skills which can be readily adapted to the needs of the community. Above all, continuing responsibility and the personal professional relationship between a general practitioner and his patient demand that physical, psychological and social factors should be part of any behavioural statement we might produce.

In this context it is hard to improve on the words of Professor E. Kass, who accused the profession of being too disease orientated because we tend to consider urinary tract infection only in terms of renal failure:

The effect of bacteriuria as a cause of absence from school or from work needs more direct measurement. Observations on the absentee records of schoolgirls during the years preceding the discovery of their bacteriuria would be a useful approach to determining whether bacteriuria had an adverse effect on daily lives. It is more difficult to gauge the emotional impact of the teaching that sexual activity is a determinant of bacteriuria. One suspects that there is more personal unhappiness and marital discord arising from this teaching than is immediately obvious. The key point is that we address ourselves to determining the impact of chronic disorders such as bacteriuria on a broader life experience and not limit ourselves to one or other selected end point that happens to be of particular interest.[6]

It is not without interest that an eminent professor of bacteriology who gave his name to the concept of significant bacteriuria should support ideas which embody current thinking about general practice.

Table 5.4   The general practitioner. A job definition

The general practitioner is a licensed medical graduate who gives personal primary and continuing care to individuals, families and a practice population, irrespective of age, sex and illness. It is the synthesis of these functions which is unique. He will attend his patients in his consulting room and in their homes and sometimes in a clinic or hospital. His aim is to make early diagnoses. He will include and integrate physical, psychological and social factors in his considerations about health and illness. This will be expressed in the care of his patients. He will make an initial decision about every problem which is presented to him as a doctor. He will undertake the continuing management of his patients with chronic, recurrent or terminal illness. Prolonged contact means that he can use repeated opportunities to gather information at a pace appropriate to each patient and build up a relationship of trust which he can use professionally. He will practise in co-operation with other colleagues, medical and non-medical. He will know how and when to intervene through treatment, prevention and education to promote the health of his patients and their families. He will recognize that he also has a professional responsibility to the community.

Joint Committee for Postgraduate Training in General Practice, European Working Party, Leeuwenhorst (RCGP, 1974)

TERMINOLOGY AND DEFINITIONS

One of the most difficult tasks in medicine is to produce an adequate definition of any disease; if one assumes that a definition must include a set of criteria which are fulfilled by all persons said to have the disease and no one without it, the task is probably impossible. Nevertheless, this task must be attempted if learning, teaching, audit and research are to proceed. The Medical Research Council Bacteriuria Committee have suggested the following clinical and bacteriological definitions[7].

(1) *Urinary tract infection:* The presence of micro-organisms in the urinary tract

(2) *Bacteriuria:* The presence of bacteria in bladder urine. For epidemiological purposes this may be detected by quantitative urine culture; its presence is usually indicated by the finding of 100 000 colony forming units (cfu) per ml of freshly voided urine and any growth from urine obtained by suprapubic aspiration. In infants the aspiration needle may occasionally be advanced into the rectum, resulting in a false positive culture; this can be recognized as the cause of a positive culture when urine is aspirated on withdrawal rather than advancement of the needle

(3) *Bladder bacteriuria:* The presence of bacteria in urine obtained from the bladder by catheter or by suprapubic aspiration

(4) *Covert bacteriuria:* Significant bacteriuria detected by the screening of apparently healthy populations. This term is preferred to 'asymptomatic significant' bacteriuria

(5) *Upper tract bacteriuria:* The presence of bacteria in urine collected from the renal pelvis or ureter(s) or both. This may indicate renal infection, but in the presence of vesico-ureteric reflux the organism may derive from the bladder

(6) *Frequency and dysuria syndrome:* A clinical syndrome often called cystitis (especially by lay people) consisting of frequency and dysuria. Bladder bacteriuria may or may not be present

(7) *Bacterial cystitis:* A syndrome consisting of dysuria and frequency of micturition by day and night. Bladder bacteriuria is present and is usually associated with pyuria and sometimes haematuria

(8) *Abacterial cystitis:* A syndrome consisting of frequency and dysuria in the absence of bladder bacteriuria. The term 'urethral syndrome', previously applied to this category of patient, is not now recommended because there is no evidence of urethral disease in most patients

(9) *Acute bacterial pyelonephritis:* A syndrome consisting of loin pain, tenderness and pyrexia accompanied by bacteriuria, bacteraemia, pyuria and sometimes haematuria. The condition is associated with bacterial infection of the kidney

(10) *Response:* Disappearance of bacteriuria after treatment

(11) *Relapse:* Post-treatment recurrence of bacteriuria due to the same organism as that originally isolated. Relapse of infection usually occurs within 6 weeks of cessation of treatment

(12) *Persistent infection:* Bacteriuria persisting during and after treatment

(13) *Reinfection:* Recurrence of bacteriuria after treatment due to an organism different from that originally isolated. Reinfection with the same organism cannot be differentiated from relapse

(14) *Criteria for cure:* In all treatment trials these should be carefully defined. Urine specimens should be collected at specified times after completion of treatment over a defined period (not usually less than 6 weeks). If the follow-up specimens show no evidence of infection or if reinfection is found, the subject is considered to have been cured of the original infection. If the post-treatment specimens show a relapse or if bacteriuria persists, treatment may be deemed to have failed

EPIDEMIOLOGY AND PRESENTATION IN GENERAL PRACTICE

The general practitioner meets four types of patient with urinary symptoms. These are (1) women with the dysuria and frequency syndrome, (2) men with essentially similar symptoms often referred to as 'prostatitis', (3) children and (4) the elderly. Diagnostic criteria and management norms need to vary within each subgroup, for reasons outlined below.

The incidence of symptomatic urinary infection in women, men and children in general practice is about two per 1000 patients at risk per year by the Kass Criterion (significant bacteriuria). This means that the practitioner with an average list size can expect 30–40 patients each year whose symptoms are accompanied by significant bacteriuria. As many again may present with symptoms strongly suggesting infection, but on bacteriological investigation of a urine specimen significant bacteriuria is not isolated. Table 5.1 presents the incidence of urinary symptoms and urinary infection by the Kass Criterion in women, men and children in the author's practice. It should be remembered that there will be some interpractice variation reflecting different interests in various practitioners, the practice administration and the patients themselves. Table 5.5 presents the prevalence of 'covert bacteriuria' in various subgroups in the community.

Table 5.5 Prevalence of covert bacteriuria in different groups

Group	Prevalence %	Comment
Neonates	1	M:F 3:1 ratio
Infants and schoolchildren		
Boys	0.2	
Girls	0.8	
Primary school		
Girls	1.6	
Boys	0.4	
Adult women	4	
Adult men	0.5	
Pregnant women	4.0	
The elderly (over 65)		
Women	21	
Men	19	

Women with the dysuria and frequency syndrome

These form the largest category of patient which we meet in general practice. There is an incidence of about 48 per 1000 women over the age of 15 each year if cystitis symptoms alone are used as diagnostic criteria. Of particular relevance, however, is the fact that only half of them have significant bacteriuria when their urines are cultured and that a careful history will not predict the result.

Our overall aim must be to define the problem(s) accurately enough to prepare an acceptable management plan. Women with the dysuria and frequency syndrome are not a homogenous group. About one third of women presenting during a 12-month period are experiencing their very first attack of symptoms. The majority of the remainder have had previous attacks on two or three occasions and a small minority get frequently recurring and distressing attacks of symptoms which seriously interfere with daily living. The majority of women present with infrequent attacks and a few constitutional symptoms, some have frequent attacks but few constitutional symptoms and a few have severe constitutional symptoms suggesting acute pyelonephritis. Each group requires a different approach. Young women are particularly likely to present with their first attack which may reflect sexual activity and may be associated with feelings of guilt, anxiety about a pregnancy and about the possibility of venereal disease or concern that they might be developing a problem which could interfere with their sexual life. This history should allow patient ideas to be expressed, providing an opportunity for contraception counselling. It is doubtful whether anything is to be gained by a physical examination unless the patient requests one.

Women who have frequent attacks but few constitutional symptoms require a different approach, not least in importance being sympathy, interest and an active desire to help. The history should be detailed in order to explore any precipitating factors, as managing these constitutes an approach to prophylaxis (Table 5.6). It is important to allow the patient to express the effect of her problem on her daily and personal life, especially if she is coming to believe that sex makes her ill. Physical examination (abdomen and

Table 5.6 Precipitating factors possibly implicated in recurrent attacks of the dysuria and frequency syndrome and some management suggestions

Precipitating factors	Management
Sexual intercourse	Scrupulous hygiene. Lubricants. Bladder emptying after intercourse. Alternative positions. Pillow under buttocks. Nitrofurantoin 50 mg after intercourse. Psychosexual history
Psychological stress	Counselling. Psychosexual history. Consider short course of a sedative, or if indicated antidepressive therapy
Cold weather	Warm underclothing. Trousers rather than skirts or dresses
Allergies	Psychosexual history. Avoid known allergens. Consider antihistamines or desensitization
Menopause	Psychosexual history. Dienoestrol pessaries, 1 nocte for 1 week every 3 months. Dienoestrol cream. Pentovis capsules 2 b.d. for 2 weeks
Menstruation	Scrupulous hygiene. A simple diuretic for a few days before a period starts. Trial of oral contraceptives

pelvis) is advisable if only to reassure the patient that all is well. It is unlikely that relevant pathology will be discovered. When symptoms of dysuria and frequency are accompanied by loin pain and rigors and marked constitutional symptoms, it is clearly necessary to enquire about previous attacks of pyelonephritis and to palpate for renal tenderness.

Drug treatment

There is an analogy between the dysuria and frequency syndrome and sore throats. We know that most throat infections are viral in aetiology yet we do not swab all throats. We use clinical criteria to determine whether or not we will prescribe penicillin, recognizing that bacteriological investigation is not particularly helpful. We may give aspirin to some streptococcal throats, but it hardly matters because most patients will get better anyway and complications are unlikely; if penicillin is given to some viral throats there is no real harm done. Similarly, we know that half the women with symptoms will not have significant bacteriuria and, if we treat all with symptoms, some women may get unnecessary treatment. However, many women with symptoms and significant bacteriuria will get better without antibacterial therapy. It seems very reasonable to give short courses of antibacterial treatment to all with moderately severe symptoms. Women with mild symptoms can be given analgesics and encouraged to further the activity of their own natural defence mechanisms by drinking plenty of fluids. There is no doubt that short courses of treatment are to be preferred. A 3-day course of amoxycillin is no less effective than a 10-day course[8] and the same probably holds true for all antibiotics used in the management of urinary tract infection. The choice of drug should be based on safety, effectiveness and cost. Resistance patterns should ideally be discussed with local microbiology laboratories. Currently recommended single dose regimens include a single dose of 400 mg trimethoprim or four tablets of co-trimoxazole (320 mg of trimethoprim with 1600 mg sulphonamide) or a suspension of 3 g amoxycillin to be taken last thing before bed at night. An alternative approach is co-trimoxazole two tablets at night for three nights. If tissue infection (e.g. pyelonephritis) is suspected, a bactericidal drug (such as ampicillin) is preferable to a bacteriostatic drug (such as a sulphonamide) and treatment should be given for a full 7 days.

Women with frequent attacks can be considerably improved by prophylactic antibacterial therapy. They can be given a supply of tablets prophylactically, for example, nitrofurantoin 50 mg nocte after intercourse or other recognized provoking situations. Alternatively, a regular 3–6 month course of this drug or trimethoprim one tablet nocte can be advised.

Follow-up

There is no evidence that recurrent infection in women leads to rise in blood pressure, serum urea concentration or kidney scarring. Nevertheless, despite adequate therapy and bacteriological cure, nearly one third of women with symptoms and significant bacteriuria will develop significant bacteriuria again over a 3-month follow-up and only half of these will have symptoms. This is of little significance unless symptoms are troublesome. Routine follow-up is unnecessary for most women unless infection is associated with pregnancy, known kidney damage or frequent attacks.

Referral

Table 5.2 demonstrates the referral pattern of general practitioners in the United Kingdom.

There is no doubt that far too many women have been subjected to unpleasant investigations (excretion urography or cystourethroscopy) as a result of anxieties about deteriorating renal function. Women with clinical evidence of pyelonephritis require excretion urography and patients with atypical features such as haematuria will require further investigation. Women with frequent distressing attacks may require referral to an interested specialist for investigation of the lower urinary tract in order to assess bladder function and urethral flow properties.

The commonly stated advice that patients with a second or third attack require investigation is overscrupulous.

The adult male

Symptoms suggesting urinary tract infection are responsible for ten consultations each year per 1000 men at risk. The incidence of bacteriologically confirmed urinary infection in this group is four per 1000. The incidence of symptoms and infection increases with age, owing to prostate hypertrophy which impairs defence mechanisms. Bacteria can multiply in prostate fluid as well as urine and as prostate fluid contains an antibacterial substance, organism counts could be low for this reason and low counts cannot be assumed necessarily to be due to contamination. There is often a marked tissue response in men and symptoms may be pronounced.

Older men may present primarily with mild obstruction symptoms such as hesitancy, urgency and an altered urine stream.

Other men present primarily with symptoms suggesting infection such as dysuria and frequency, haematuria, offensive urine, mild rigors or loin pain. Yet another group presents with vague symptoms such as low back pain and perineal discomfort and mild micturition disturbances, and occasionally flu-like symptoms predominate. The history should allow for psychosexual problems and examination should include palpation of the testicles and epididymis for evidence of local spread of infection as well as rectal examination of the prostate gland and bladder palpation to detect subacute or chronic obstruction. It is rather embarrassing to be told by a grinning partner that your antibiotics did not help Mr Brown at all and as he had a bladder up to his umbilicus he was sent into hospital!

There is a close relationship between bladder urine infection, prostatitis and posterior urethritis and it is seldom easy and fairly pointless to try and separate the three, which may often co-exist. Organisms may multiply in prostatic fluid which may contain Prostatic Antibacterial Factor (PAF), and this may be one reason why infection within the urinary tract is less common in men. The usual explanation given – that women have a shorter urethra – is not really very convincing. Why don't small mammals get overwhelming infection? Urine culture may be helpful and may reveal significant bacteriuria, smaller numbers of organisms or may be sterile; the Kass Criterion is of limited value as any number of organisms may be relevant.

The first priority in management is to eradicate infection. The concentration of most agents active against Gram-negative organisms is considerably less in the prostate than the plasma, and because of this co-trimoxazole or trimethoprim alone may be preferred in a dosage of two tablets, twice daily for 10 days. Referral of the patient, preferably to a urological surgeon, is advisable in all men with symptoms, the only exception perhaps being the young man with an isolated attack who tends not to have an underlying lesion. An excretion urogram is mandatory and often reveals a prostate filling defect in the bladder associated with a residual urine. Such investigations can be ordered from the practice while awaiting a urological opinion. Of 26 consecutive men with symptoms referred to a consultant urologist in the author's practice, five required prostatectomy and a further two had laparotomies because of upper tract lesions. Follow-up in the practice, including urine assessment, is usually indicated.

The child

The incidence of urinary infection in childhood using a single dip slide with significant bacteriuria is 7.7 per 1000 girls at risk and 3.8 per 1000 boys at risk per year.

Urinary infection matters in children, particularly in infants and preschool children. This is because, in this group of patients, infection has been shown to lead to renal scarring in the presence of vesico-ureteric reflux. Indeed, the chance finding of scarred kidneys in adult life is an indication that infection occurred in early childhood.

Two factors complicate diagnosis. First, contamination is common, particularly in neonates, and as vague symptoms of dysuria and frequency in children are not uncommon, infection can easily be said to exist when it doesn't. Second, especially in preschool children, genuine urinary infection may produce vague systemic symptoms such as pyrexia of unknown origin (PUO) and vague abdominal pain rather than urinary symptoms. The above observations emphasize the importance of adequate investigation facilities in general practice. It is unthinkable that infants and children should receive traumatic micturating cystograms and cystoscopies simply because they have vague dysuria and provide a contaminated specimen. Conversely, it would be a tragedy if kidney scarring should continue to occur in the presence of reflux that could be identified if appropriate referrals had been made. If dip slides are incubated in the practice and significant bacteriuria is discovered, they could be posted to the laboratory for identification of the pathogens and sensitivity studies. As in adults, *Escherichia coli* is the predominant pathogen, but proteus infection is ten times commoner in boys. Care should be taken in collecting the specimen. As so much depends on the diagnosis, suprapubic aspiration might be considered, especially in infants and preschool children. The technique is simple and no more hazardous than a venepuncture; the abdominal skin is cleansed with a plain water swab and using a 4 cm (1½ inch) (green) needle and a 10 cc syringe the abdomen is penetrated in the midline about 4 cm (1½ inches) above the symphysis, withdrawing the needle on entry rather than on the way out. Complications are extremely rare.

The abdomen should be examined and the renal area palpated; the blood pressure should be checked.

Treatment is usually with co-trimoxazole, trimethoprim alone, or ampicillin for a period of at least 10 days.

All children with urinary tract infections require radiological investigation, initially at least an excretion urogram. When regular follow-up is carried out in general practice, it would seem reasonable to refer a child for more traumatic micturating cystography and other investigations if recurrent bacteriuria is demonstrated or if excretion urography has revealed an abnormal tract. Children under 2 years are particularly at risk for scarring and should be referred for full investigation straight away. In ideal circumstances, referral should be to a nephrologist or urologist with a particular interest in paediatric problems and time should be spent talking with the mother to give her an opportunity to discuss her anxieties. The admission to hospital of a young child, particularly when traumatic investigations are to be carried out, can have a profound effect on mother–child relationships. All this is especially true in relation to kidney disease, as the kidneys are second only to the heart as a cause of fears about long term health.

Thorough investigation will result in four categories of patient: children with no apparent abnormality, children with reflux and no scarring, children with reflux and scarring and children with congenital abnormalities other than reflux, some of which, e.g. urethral valves, may be surgically correctable. Reflux is always abnormal. If marked, surgical correction may be advised, but conservative treatment with long term low dose antibiotic prophylaxis is usually tried first. In the author's (DB) practice (7800 patients) 20 children are currently receiving follow-up. Four have had bilateral ureteric re-implants and one has had a pyeloplasty.

Mothers of children with scarred kidneys are reminded that the vast majority of people with scarred kidneys do very well indeed and that we do not know what causes scarred kidneys to fail.

The elderly

Urinary symptoms are common in the elderly. The possibility that infection might be associated with incontinence, and vague symptoms such as PUO and confusion, emphasize that bacteriological examination of the urine is frequently required. However, urinary incontinence is often the cause rather than the result of urinary infection since it interferes with defence mechanisms against ascending infection. In any individual patient, it is often difficult to differentiate between acute bacteriuria causing symptoms and chronic bacteriuria which may be asymptomatic or associated with symptoms from a third cause. A trial of therapy is often the only satisfactory assessment. If symptoms disappear, further episodes merit treatment.

Bacteriuria in the elderly in general practice is a benign problem and has no significance in terms of deteriorating renal function. There is little justification for routine bacteriological examination of urine from elderly patients with indwelling catheters. Infection is inevitable, but it is of little relevance unless symptoms intervene.

SCREENING FOR BACTERIURIA

The consensus view at present is that, because of the difficulties involved in getting clean catch specimens from the group of patients most likely to benefit from the procedure and in view of the fact that we do not know what causes scarred kidneys to fail, screening cannot be recommended in the United Kingdom. Considerable anxiety would be induced in the parents of the many children who would be found to have normal urinary tracts and contaminated specimens. The only indication for screening in general practice is in the ante-natal clinic when treatment of asymptomatic bacteriuric women with a 7-day course of ampicillin will prevent the possible later development of acute pyelonephritis.

REFERENCES

1. Waters, W. E. (1969). Prevalence of symptoms of urinary tract infection in women. *Brt. J. Prev. Soc. Med.*, **23**, 263–6

2. Walker, M., Heady, J. A. and Shader, A. G.(1983). The prevalence of dysuria in women in London. *J. R. Coll. Gen. Practit.*, **33**, 411–15
3. Fry, J., Dilane, J. B., Joiner, C. I. and Williams, J. D. (1962). Acute urinary infections, their course and outcome in general practice with special reference to chronic pyelonephritis. *Lancet*, **1**, 1318–21
4. Review (1968). Management of patients with upper or lower urinary tract infection. *Br. Med. J.*, **3**, 600–2
5. Asscher, A. W. (1978). Management of frequency and dysuria. *Br. Med. J.*, **1**, 1531–3
6. Kass, E. H. (1979). Epidemiologic aspects of infections of the urinary tract. In Kass, E. H. and Brumfitt, W. (eds.) *Infections of the Urinary Tract*. (Chicago: University of Chicago Press)
7. Medical Research Council Bacteriuria Committee (1979). Recommended terminology of urinary tract infections. *Br. Med. J.*, **2**, 717–9
8. Charlton, C. A. C., Crowther, A., Davies, J. G., Dynes, J., Haward, M. W. A., Mann, P. G. and Rye, S. (1976). Three-day and ten-day chemotherapy for urinary tract infections in general practice. *Br. Med. J.*, **1**, 124–6

6

Vaginal Discharge and Pelvic Infection

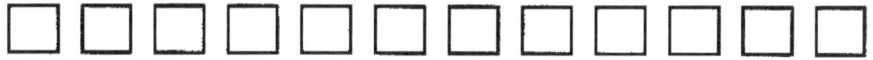

PRESENTATION

In the days when consultants were allowed, if not expected, to be male chauvinists, an eminent Manchester gynaecologist used to tell his patients in front of the students that if they did not have a vaginal discharge they would squeak when they walked! Today such behaviour would rightly be regarded as a 'put down'.

The story does illustrate, however, that when a woman complains of a vaginal discharge her ideas about the problem may be different from, if not totally incompatible with, traditional medical ideas about it, and that in general practice it may be even more important to identify and work with the patient's ideas than simply to display painfully acquired knowledge about vaginal pathogens and their epidemiological behaviour.

The size of the problem

In 1982 in DB's practice there were 82 new episodes of 'vaginal discharge'. This represents 0.7% of all first episodes of illness in the practice and 2% of first episodes of infection. This means that, on our figures, in a practice of 2500 patients 26 women will consult their general practitioner each year with a vaginal discharge, a figure which compares well with Fry's experience of 30 such patients each year.

Some data about presentation in general practice

Fry found that when his 30 patients were investigated no cause was found in 18 of them (60%). Ten women (33%) had a candida vaginitis and two women (7%) had a trichomonal infection. Veneral disease was rare, gonorrhoea occurring only once every 4–5 years.

This is the experience of most general practitioners but it is contrary to the experience of most gynaecological outpatient clinics. The reason is often said to be better investigation facilities in the hospital, but a more likely explanation lies in the nature of the problem and the effect of the referral system. Women react differently to the presence of a discharge. Some will tolerate a copious and offensive discharge while others will not accept slight staining. In today's society with its vaginal deodorants and panty liners the advertisers' 'target' is not prepared to accept departure from the aseptic, white and pure ideal she is led to believe is the norm.

THE CAUSES

A vaginal discharge then may be physiological, inflammatory or due to a specific vaginal pathogen (Table 6.1). *Physiological* causes may include a normally functioning vaginal epithelium, excessive secretions associated with a simple cervical erosion, the changes of early pregnancy and atrophic (oestrogen deficient) vaginitis. *Inflammatory* causes include retained tampons, self-prescribed agents such as douches, female deodorants and antiseptic substances in the bath water. Most vaginal infections are due to *Candida albicans, Trichomonas vaginalis, Herpesvirus hominis, Chlamydia trachomatus* and *Neisseria gonorrhoeae*. Recent work suggests that *Gardnerella vaginalis* (previously *Haemophilus vaginalis*) may be responsible, possibly in association with anaerobes such as *bacteroides* spp. and peptococci which may be implicated in mixed infections.

Table 6.1 Causes of vaginal discharge

Physiological
   Cervical ectropian
   Pregnancy
   Oestrogen deficiency (atrophic vaginitis)

Inflammatory
   Douches
   Deodorants
   Bath salts, perfumes etc

Pathological
   Candida spp
   Trichomonas vaginalis
   Gardnerella (Haemophilus) vaginalis
   Chlamydia spp.
   Neisseria gonorrhoeae
   Treponema pallidum
   ? Anaerobic organisms

CLINICAL FEATURES

When a vaginal discharge is due to a specific vaginal pathogen it may well be possible to identify the causative organism on clinical grounds.

Monilial vaginitis

Genital candidosis has been increasing steadily over the last decade, probably due to the increasing use of broad spectrum antibiotics and possibly oral contraceptives. In 90–95% of cases, *Candida albicans* is the responsible organism. It is a yeast-like organism which causes monilial vaginitis or thrush. The vaginal discharge is usually thick, whitish and cheesy in consistency and is associated with intense vulval and vaginal pruritus, especially in association with pregnancy or diabetes mellitus. The vulval skin may be bluish-red, scaly, oedematous and sore and in a few cases examination may be very painful indeed.

Trichomonas vaginitis

Trichomonas vaginalis is a flagellate protozoa which can be identified microscopically by means of a wet slide preparation under dark ground illumination. Culture is more accurate and an orientated and interested cytologist examining cervical or vaginal smears is probably equally effective. The organism produces a vaginal discharge with vaginitis. The discharge may be frothy, malodorous and purulent and associated with vulval oedema, pruritus and intertrigo. Not infrequently there may be only a mild discharge which can be ignored by the patient. On speculum examination the vaginal walls may be inflamed and the cervix inflamed and speckled.

Other organisms

Genital herpes

Infections are usually caused by *Herpesvirus hominis* and they are usually sexually transmitted. There is no effective remedy and there is a suspicion that the organism may be oncogenic. The diagnosis is usually made when vesicles are seen on the cervix but they only appear during the first few days. The infection usually settles down but may well recur.

Gardnerella

Non-specific vaginitis due to gardnerella in combination with anaerobes may be common in general practice.

Gonorrhoea and syphilis

Gonorrhoea and syphilis are rare indeed in this context but should always be borne in mind in women between 15 and 24, women travelling abroad and unmarried women who may be particularly at risk (see Chapter 7).

AN APPROACH TO DIAGNOSIS

Women who present with vaginal discharge in general practice are very largely between the ages of 15 and 45 and are sexually active (Figure 6.1). Perhaps the most important first step is to ensure

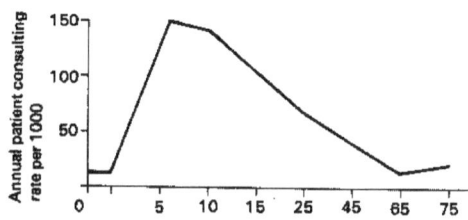

Figure 6.1   Vaginal discharge – age prevalence (RCGP/OPCS 1974)

that the patient feels at ease, especially if she is presenting her problem to a male doctor. The patient must be allowed to relate her story in her own way without interruption from the doctor, including the effects of the problem on her feelings about herself and on her sexual life.

A vaginal examination (speculum and bimanual) should always be offered but never pressed, as the nature of the discharge will often be a guide to the predominant organism (mixed infections are possible.) Other advantages are that discharge due to forgotten tampons, cervical polyps and erosions, carcinoma of the cervix and secondarily infected atrophic vaginitis will be apparent, as will intrauterine causes and pelvic inflammatory disease. The appearance of the discharge may well be characteristic. If the vagina is clean and healthy, do not give the patient the impression that she is disbelieved. She may have noticed a physiological discharge and be unduly anxious, for example about the behaviour of a sexual partner, or she may well have had a bath only hours before. It is often surprising, although always understandable, how before a medical examination so many women attempt to remove the discharge they have noticed!

An attempt should be made to identify a causative organism, especially if the appearance of the discharge is unhelpful. A cervical smear can be taken and a high vaginal swab immersed in Stuart's transport medium. If gonorrhoea is suspected, high vag-

91

inal swabs, urethral swabs, cervical swabs and rectal swabs should all be immersed in Stuart's transport medium and posted to the laboratory. Light microscopy of a saline suspension of vaginal secretions using 10% potassium hydroxide and warming to lyse other cellular elements is helpful in monilia vaginitis, but culture is the more accurate procedure. Repeated examinations may sometimes be necessary, especially with trichomonas infection. Gram-staining is helpful when looking for monilia. Oral gram-positive yeast-like forms and mycelia are looked for in the smear.

THE MANAGEMENT APPROACH

Management will depend crucially on whether patient and doctor together have come to the conclusion that the diagnosis is physiological or pathological.

If the former, physiological, diagnosis is likely, the main management aim will be to enable the patient to air her anxieties and to learn something about her own body function.

If the condition is probably pathological, a decision must be made whether to take a sexual history and whether to offer treatment to the male partner. In this context, the general practitioner's prior relationship with and knowledge of his patient is of inestimable value.

TREATMENT OF TRICHOMONAS INFECTIONS

Gaya and Hawkins state that over the past two decades the management of trichomoniasis has been bedevilled by three statements of questionable validity which have been repeated over the years.

The first of these statements is that trichomonal infection is *always sexually transmitted.* General practitioners who have treated the infection in Caesar's wife (not to mention a partner's wife) have always found it difficult to live with this concept. The infection occurs in nuns and in women isolated from sexual contact in mental institutions. Moreover, it is undoubtedly transmitted by vaginal speculae. Indeed many studies have shown that the infection is commoner in women who reattend gynaecological outpatients than in women making their first visit! A fair summary of the evidence is that trichomonal infection is often sexually transmitted.

The second unsubstantiated dictum is that patients with trichomonas *commonly have gonorrhoea as well*. It is true that almost half the patients attending venereal disease clinics with trichomonas have gonorrhoea as well, but this figure falls to under 5% in gynaecological outpatient clinics and antental clinics and to less than 1% in general practice.

The final concept that appears to be losing ground is that the *sexual consort should always be treated if recurrence is to be prevented*. In most cases *T. vaginalis* has only a very limited survival in the male partner.

The introduction of oral metronidazole (Flagyl) revolutionized the management of vaginal trichomoniasis when it first appeared 20 years ago, and it is still the treatment of choice. Standard treatment is 200 mg t.d.s. orally after food for 7 days, together with advice to avoid alcohol while taking the tablets and to avoid sexual intercourse for 2 weeks. No strains of trichomonas resistant to metronidazole have yet been isolated from humans and treatment is effective in over 80% (Table 6.2).

Side-effects include gastrointestinal disturbances, headaches, dizziness and skin eruptions.

Treatment failures

Treatment failures (25%) are due to failure to take the drug regularly, failure of absorption from the intestine or reinfection by a sexual contact. The best approach is to assume *failure to take the drug regularly* and give a single large dose of 2 g with a drink of fruit juice. *Suspected reinfection* can be dealt with by giving a repeated 10-day course to patient and consort. Failure yet again gives rise to suspicion of *malabsorption* and requires the use of an increased oral dose (2 g daily in divided doses for 3 days) or combined oral and vaginal administration using Flagyl suppositories by the latter route. Nimorazole (Naxogin) 250 mg b.d. for 6 days is a useful alternative to metronidazole and a new intro-

Table 6.2   Treatment of vaginal discharge

Candidosis
Nystatin cream to vulva
Nystatin pessaries (100 000 units) 1 or 2 intravaginally nocte for 14 days
Nystatin tablets (500 000 units) 1 t.d.s. orally for 10 days to prevent
  reinfection
or
Candicidin ointment to vulva
Candicidin tablets 3 mg 1 b.d. intravaginally for 14 days
or
Clotrimazole cream to vulva
Clotrimazole vaginal tablets 100 mg 2 nocte for 3 days or 1 nocte for 6
  days

Trichomonas and gardnerella
Metronidazole 200 mg t.d.s. for 7 days orally
or
Metronidazole 2 g stat. orally (avoid alcohol)
or
Nimorazole 250 mg b.d. for 6 doses orally
or
Nimorazole 2 g stat. orally (avoid alcohol)

duction, tinidazole (Fasigyn), marketed for the prophylaxis and
treatment of anaerobic infections awaits evaluation.

TREATMENT OF MONILIAL VAGINITIS

Nystatin (Nystan) is more effective than gentian violet and there
is no evidence that any of the newer agents such as candicidin
(Candeptin) and miconazole (Daktarin) are more effective.

Standard treatment is (according to severity) with one or two
nystatin pessaries each containing 100 000 units inserted into the
vaginal vault each night for a fortnight, together with the local
application of nystatin cream for vulval irritation (Table 6.2). The
patient should be urged to complete the treatment and to wash
her hands after insertion of the pessaries to prevent nail infection.
She should be warned that clothes may be stained yellow!

Treatment failures

Recurrence, or treatment failures, should be treated with pro-longed courses over several weeks using a slowly decreasing dose. If this fails it is necessary to ensure that the problem is candidiasis and to stop all treatment until a positive culture is obtained. Lactic acid pessaries and 0.5% hydrocortisone cream may be used until a firm diagnosis is made. If the diagnosis is confirmed, a full course of pessaries and cream should be repeated together with oral nystatin 500 000 units t.d.s. for 10 days to prevent reinfection of the vagina from the gut. Another approach is to use nystatin pessaries regularly for three consecutive nights each month. If the consort has noticed irritation he should be examined and treated, and treatment may be required for associated cervical erosions. It may be necessary to try an alternative form of contraception if the 'pill' is incriminated in a treatment failure.

DRUG TREATMENT OF INFECTION WITH OTHER ORGANISMS

Non-specific vaginitis due to gardnerella in combination with anaerobes gives a satisfactory response to metronidazole (Table 6.2). The drug may work through both its activity against anaerobes and its specific action against *G. vaginitis*. Povidone-iodine (Betadine) pessaries are a useful though messy vaginal an-tiseptic agent. Alternatives include penotrane (Hydrargaphen) pes-saries and SVC effervescent vaginal tablets.

Postmenopausal women may sometimes develop a secondary Gram-negative bacterial vaginitis which is offensive and purulent and which responds to neomycin sulphate (Tampovagan N) pes-saries.

PELVIC INFAMMATORY DISEASE

Most cases of pelvic inflammatory disease are caused by ascending infection and most are associated with sexual activity. Hospital admissions for both acute and chronic pelvic inflammatory disease increased by 8.7% a year among women aged 15–44 in England

and Wales between 1966 and 1976 (Figure 6.2). Although hospital admissions for chronic disease are increasing more rapidly than for acute disease, the latter was three times as common as chronic disease. Peak incidence of acute disease is at age 20–24 and of chronic at 25–29.

Hospital admissions represent only a small fraction of the disease in the community; less than 10% of cases referred to outpatient clinics are admitted to hospital. Rates for both acute and chronic pelvic inflammatory disease are highest among divorced women. At all ages married women have higher rates for chronic disease than single women.

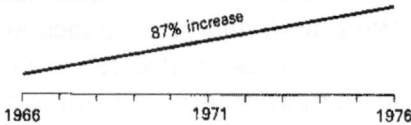

1966   1971   1976

Figure 6.2 Hospital admission for both acute and chronic pelvic inflammatory disease

The cause

Pelvic inflammatory disease is clearly one of the many increasingly recognized 'perils' of permissiveness. All women using an IUCD have an increased risk of pelvic infection. Pathogenic organisms may be difficult to grow by ordinary bacteriological techniques. This applies both to the anaerobic organisms now recognized as important secondary invaders, and to *Chlamydia trachomatis* which is important as a primary pathogen.

Chlamydia is an intracellular organism present in about 5% of asymptomatic women. The incidence of antichlamydial antibodies found in acute salpingitis was 72% in one reported series compared with 10% of controls without salpingitis.

Clinical features

Pain is a prominent feature; it is often felt across the lower abdomen and may radiate to the back. It may be aggravated by movement, micturition, defecation or intercourse. In severe infection there may be malaise, vomiting and rigors. The patient may look flushed and ill, in pain, and may have guarding and rebound tenderness. On bimanual examination there is tenderness which in severe cases amounts to cervical excitation. The condition may need to be differentiated from appendicitis, ectopic pregnancy, ovarian cyst, endometriosis and occasionally tuberculosis. Laparoscopy may be indicated if there is doubt about the diagnosis or if symptoms do not improve within 24 hours of starting treatment.

Management

Many patients with pelvic inflammatory disease may be treated at home but patients who fail to respond to treatment may need hospital referral, possibly after a domiciliary consultation with a consultant gynaecologist. Patients who have severe pain, perhaps associated with constitutional symptoms, will require prompt admission.

Ampicillin in a dosage of 250 mg q.i.d. for 10 days is a good choice of drug in acute cases. For less acute infections tetracycline is a good choice, as it is active against chlamydia. Whichever drug is used it is now accepted practice to give metronidazole (Flagyl) at the same time, as this is active against the anaerobic organisms which are so often involved in secondary infection.

THE NEED FOR HOSPITAL REFERRAL

Very few patients with a vaginal discharge should need hospital referral. They will include the women whose discharge is secondary to some primary uterovaginal pathology and some women with recurrent vaginal infection who are suspected to have atypical or obscure pathogens. Tuberculosis should always be considered in immigrant women from the Indian subcontinent.

Attacks of acute pelvic infection may resolve completely or proceed to pyosalpinx, tubo-ovarian abscess, subacute or chronic salpingitis, hydrosalpinx or pelvic adhesions. As a result the patient may be completely asymptomatic with functioning tubes and with fertility unimpaired; she may be symptomless and subfertile or she may have chronic pain and further acute exacerbations. Further medical treatment may include bed rest, antibiotics, anti-inflammatory agents, pelvic short wave diathermy and occasionally surgery.

REFERENCES AND FURTHER READING

Budden, G. C. (1982). Pelvic inflammatory disease *Update*, **24** (12), 2429

Gaya, D. and Hawkins, D. F. (1981). Pelvic infection. In Hawkins, D. F. (ed.) *Gynaecological Therapeutics* (London: Baillière Tindall)

Fry, J. (1983). *Common Diseases: Their Nature, Incidence and Care*. 3rd Edn (Lancaster: MTP Press)

RCGP/OPCS (Office of Population Censuses and Surveys) (1974). *Studies on Medical and Population Subjects. No. 26. Morbidity Statistics from General Practice. Second National Study 1970-71*. (London: HMSO)

7

Sexually Transmitted Diseases

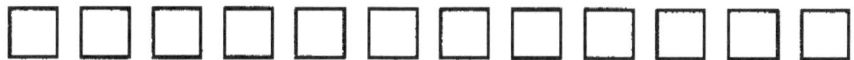

THE SIZE OF THE PROBLEM

Sexually transmitted diseases (STD) are caught by changing sexual partners and by casual sex. They could therefore be completely avoided. Paradoxically, however, they are among the commonest infectious diseases in the world. Between 1949 and 1980 the number of new cases attending NHS clinics increased fourfold (Tables 7.1, 7.2). More than one person in every 100 of the UK population is likely to attend a clinic each year. Over the period referred to, gonorrhoea and non-specific infections increased significantly whereas syphilis has declined. Most important of all, perhaps, is that an estimated 1500–2000 young women become sterile each year as a result of infection by gonorrhoea (Catterall, 1979).

The routine published statistics for sexually transmitted diseases underestimate the problem, however, since they do not include three other possible categories of patient – those in general or private practice, those in antenatal or gynaecology clinics, symptomless patients who may never be treated and patients with symptoms who decide to ignore them. Adler and colleagues (1981) estimated the contribution of these categories of patient to the

Table 7.1   New cases at NHS clinics

	1949 No.	%	1980 No.	%
Syphilis	13 000	12	4 059	1
Gonococcal	23 000	21	54 000	12
Non-specific infections	Not recorded	—	115 000	25
Other conditions requiring treatment	30 000	27	178 000	39
Other conditions not requiring treatment	45 000	40	107 000	23
Total	111 000	100	459 000	100

DHSS Health and Personal Social Services Statistics, England (London: HMSO) 1982

total problem for gonorrhoea, trichomoniasis and candidosis (Table 7.3). The highest prevalence rates were found for candidosis, followed by trichomoniasis, with very low or zero rates for gonorrhoea.

PRESENTATION

The reasons why there has been a worldwide increase in sexually transmitted diseases must be speculative, but any list must include changes in sexual attitudes and behaviour, education, homosexuality, the contraceptive pill, social mobility, the asymptomatic carrier state and insensitivity to antibiotics.

Changes in sexual attitudes and behaviour

Sexually transmitted diseases are not acquired by couples who keep to the same partner. There is much evidence that young people are having their first sexual experience earlier and premarital sex and changing of sexual partners no longer attracts public

Table 7.2 Sexually transmitted disease in Britain: reported new cases, 1976–80

Diagnosis	1976	1977	1978	1979	1980*
Syphilis	4 306	4 780	4 866	4 485	4 460
Gonorrhoea	65 281	65 963	63 569	61 616	60 824
Chancroid	59	49	57	49	66
Lymphogranuloma venereum	39	43	34	36	35
Granuloma inguinale	36	56	14	40	20
Non-specific genital infection	101 651	105 210	107 955	113 138	125 383
Trichomoniasis	21 903	22 145	21 732	21 222	22 312
Candidiasis	39 414	41 144	42 524	42 667	48 061
Scabies	2 749	2 562	2 589	2 391	2 603
Pubic lice	6 168	6 769	7 505	8 272	8 960
Herpes simplex	7 547	8 399	9 036	9 576	10 801
Warts	23 035	26 063	27 272	27 654	31 788
Molluscum contagiosum	954	1 019	1 026	1 030	1 232
Other treponemal disease	1 142	1 117	1 088	1 103	946
Other conditions requiring treatment	44 848	48 461	52 140	55 408	65 694
Other conditions not requiring treatment	97 491	104 539	108 596	109 050	117 087
Total new cases	418 623	438 319	450 003	457 637	500 272

* Provisional figures
Source: Sexually Transmitted Diseases Surveillance 1980. (1982). *Br. Med. J.*, **284**, 124

Table 7.3 Prevalence rates for sexually transmitted diseases per 1000 population

Population	Candidosis	Trichomoniasis	Gonorrhoea
Gynaecology (no symptoms)	78	70	4
Family Planning	36	47	0
Antenatal	83	44	3
General practice (invited to attend)	93	32	0

From: Adler, M. W., Belsey, E. M. and Rogers, J. J. (1981). *Br. Med. J.* **283**, 29 disapproval or criticism. Not only this, people are also more adventurous, and infection is commoner in the mouth and throat as a result of orogenital sex and in the rectum and anus as a result of rectal sex.

Education

Women's magazines, video, television and men's magazines in particular and the media generally have undoubtedly both stimulated sexual appetites and disseminated information about sexual matters. More has been written in the last couple of decades about orgasms (whether single or multiple) than at any other time in our history. We have sexual innovations for the A level performers (101 new ways of improving your performance), vitamins for the jaded and remedial education for those who never quite caught up. The demand by patients for treatment of sexual disorders (whether real or imagined) and the demand by practitioners that sexual medicine is a specialty in its own right (will there be an MRCP (sex)?) both bear witness to the effects of education and time in modifying our attitudes.

Unfortunately, however, the perils of permissiveness have received little attention over this period, either at home, in school or in the consulting room. In terms of improving knowledge about sexually transmitted diseases, their nature, prevention and treatment, we are still, attitudinally at least, at the stage when discreet posters were placed in corners of public toilets advertising confidential treatment at local clinics. If questions from children and young people about sexual diseases were discussed as frankly as failure of sexual performance and the need for contraception, we might begin to see some reduction in the official prevalence figures.

Homosexuality

Homosexual men are particularly at risk for syphilis, gonorrhoea, genital herpes and non-specific infection. Indeed, in the world's major cities, up to 70% of infectious syphilis and 30% of gonorrhoea occurring in men occurs in homosexuals. AIDS and hepatitis B have become increasing problems. In contrast, infection in homosexual women is low because they are rarely promiscuous and tend to remain with one partner.

The contraceptive pill

The introduction of oral contraception in the 1960s has undoubtedly contributed to the increase in sexually transmitted disease. Fear of pregnancy was a deterrent to sexual promiscuity for some. Studies have shown that women using oral contraceptives tend to have more intercourse, more sexual partners and a higher incidence of genital infections than those who are not on the pill.

Social mobility

The incidence of sexually transmitted diseases rises considerably during the summer months, with peaks during the holiday period from July to October. Young people travel from country to country, continent to continent and city to city on cheap package holidays and group travel. When people are away from home and in a new environment, both opportunity and inclination for casual sex are increased, with inevitable infection posing problems for contact tracing and treatment.

The asymptomatic carrier state

It is not always realized that women can be carriers of sexually transmitted disease for many months without being aware that they are infectious. If a woman is promiscuous very many men can become infected during this time. In general, men tend to have symptoms which are more severe and which present earlier.

Antibiotic resistance

Twenty-five years ago the majority of patients with gonorrhoea could be treated with a single injection of penicillin. In some parts of the world (particularly south-east Asia) the dosage required to produce adequate cure has increased several-fold. Some gonococcous strains produce β-lactamase and afflicted patients may not be cured and may infect others after treatment, thinking they are cured.

Summary

Patients who acquire sexually transmitted disease have sex outside a stable relationship. They tend to be young (16–25) and travel (especially abroad), and women have effective contraception. By and large, most patients (especially men) are attracted to the clinics when they believe they have STD.

WHAT ARE THE SEXUALLY TRANSMITTED DISEASES?

A whole variety of conditions is listed under this heading (Table 7.2). For the purpose of this chapter we will consider gonorrhoea, non-specific genital infection, herpes simplex, genital warts and syphilis. Each condition will be considered separately and the chapter will end with a specific account of the role of the general practitioner in diagnosis and management (see also Chapters 6 and 9).

Gonorrhoea

Gonorrhoea is one of the oldest and most widespread diseases in the world. Indeed, WHO states that it is out of control, with 250 million sufferers each year; over 60 000 new episodes were reported in the United Kingdom in 1980.

Organism and incubation period

The gonococcus is a strict parasite and cannot survive for long outside the human body. Sexual intercourse is almost always the mode of infection but accidental infection can occur during birth. The incubation period is usually between 2 and 10 days, with 3.5 days being the norm. In some women the incubation period may be 30 days or more. As many as 60% of women may be asymptomatic carriers.

Symptoms and signs

The first symptom noticed by men is often a discomfort or tingling in the urethra followed by a urethral discharge, which rapidly becomes creamy, thick and purulent. This will appear 3–5 days after exposure to infection but, if untreated, the infection can spread to the posterior urethra within a fortnight. Frequency of micturition, severe dysuria and perhaps haematuria may be noticed with, on occasion, some evidence of toxic absorption such as fever, headache and pyrexia.

Over half the infected women are asymptomatic carriers and even when symptoms are present they are usually mild. Vaginal discharge, dysuria, frequency, backache or lower abdominal pain and aching in the thighs may be noticed.

Diagnosis

Clinical examination may well be helpful in that, in the male, pus can be milked from the urethra. It must be distinguished from pus due to balanitis in the uncircumcized male. In women, inguinal lymph nodes may be palpable, the labia may be reddened and oedematous and there may be a vaginitis. If pressure is applied to the urethra under the symphysis, a small amount of pus may appear at the external urinary meatus. Inspection of the cervix and a bimanual examination are both mandatory and rectal examination with a proctoscope for evidence of proctitis is advisable.

The diagnosis of gonorrhoea is a bacteriological diagnosis, however, and depends on demonstrating the gonococcus on stained slides of material from the genital tract and growing the organism on suitable culture material (Chapter 1).

Drug treatment

Penicillin is still the treatment of choice despite the emergence of resistant strains. In 1981 the number of indigenous strains of penicillinase-producing organisms began to exceed the number of imported cases. In 1981 433 (0.76%) cases of resistant strains were noted. In 1982 the figure was 1033 (2%). Procaine penicillin by single intramuscular injection of 4·8 million units, preceded – 1 hour before – by oral probenecid 1 g, is the most popular treatment regimen and produces a cure rate of over 90%.

Alternative drugs are spectinomycin hydrochloride or kanamycin sulphate given in a single intramuscular injection of 2 g.

Oral treatment is possible. Co-trimoxazole can be given in a dose of four tablets twice daily for 4 days or 3 g of ampicillin stat. preceded by 1 g of probenecid. Successful treatment will diminish the purulent discharge within hours and the patient is usually free of symptoms within 2–3 days. Patients with local or metastatic complications are usually admitted to hospital. Follow-up tests are necessary 3–5 days after treatment, 2 weeks after treatment and finally 3 months after treatment and should be accompanied by serological tests for syphilis.

Complications

Complications in men include anterior urethritis, posterior urethritis, epididymitis and proctitis. Non-specific urethritis may appear 1–2 weeks after successful treatment for gonorrhoea in about 25% of all men who acquire gonorrhoea. Chlamydia is frequently isolated; it has a longer incubation period than gonorrhoea.

Women may develop skenitis, bartholinitis, proctitis and pelvic complications such as salpingitis, tubo-ovarian abscesses and peritonitis. About one patient in five develops salpingitis. Recurrent attacks of salpingitis are common and about 25% of all patients who have salpingitis have impaired fertility or complete sterility or may be more likely to have an ectopic pregnancy.

Both men and women may develop septicaemia and arthritis, typically involving a single large joint.

Non-specific genital infection

Non-specific genital infection is the commonest condition seen in clinics for sexually transmitted diseases in Britain, over 125 000 cases being reported in 1980. Typically the condition presents as non-specific urethritis in men.

Organism and incubation period

The name of the condition suggests that the cause of the infection is unknown, but evidence has accumulated that many cases are due to *Chlamydia trachomatis* and some may be due to *Ureaplasma urealytica* (previously *Mycoplasma hominis*). Chlamydia are present in the urethra of nearly 50% of men with non-specific urethritis and over 30% of their female sexual partners, and disappear following successful treatment. Although *U. urealytica* can be grown in about 70% of men with non-specific urethritis, the organism can also be isolated from apparently healthy people of both sexes.

Symptoms and signs

The majority of men affected complain of an acute purulent urethral discharge associated with urethral irritation. Frequency of micturition and haematuria may be noticed. Symptoms can be milder than those of gonorrhoea and the infection may be symptomless or hardly noticed by the patient.

In women the clinical manifestations are difficult to determine and the condition is often asymptomatic. If symptoms are present they may be due to existing trichomonas vaginitis or *C. albicans*. Features include slight discharge, mild dysuria and mild pelvic pain. Many women learn that they are infected via an affected consort.

Diagnosis

Clinical examination may be helpful in determining complications but the diagnosis of non-specific genital infection is a diagnosis that can only be made after all the other causes of genital infection have been excluded. Slides should be Gram-stained and culture should be taken for gonococcus, trichomonas, candida and other organisms (Chapter 1).

Drug treatment

Non-specific genital infection can be resistant to treatment and does tend to relapse even after successful treatment.

C. trachomatis is sensitive to the tetracycline group of antibiotics, best results being obtained with tetracycline oxytetracycline, chlortetracycline or spiromycin. Oxytetracycline is commonly given in a dosage of 250 mg 6-hourly for 21 days. The cure rate is 70–75%. Relapse is common and about 10% of patients have repeated relapses which may go on for several years. Patients should be advised to avoid dairy produce during drug treatment and men should avoid alcoholic drink as there is some evidence that relapses can be aborted. This restriction does not apply to women.

An alternative treatment is erythromycin in a dose of 260 mg 6-hourly for 21 days, or a combination of streptomycin and sulphonamides. Streptomycin 1g can be followed by 6 g of sulphadimidine daily in divided doses for 5 days.

Patients should be seen 1 week after completing treatment and again 2 weeks later and finally at 3 months. Physical examination and bacteriological tests are recommended.

Complications

Men may develop prostatitis, epididymitis or a urethral stricture. Women may develop bartholinitis and salpingitis. Eye infections may occur in the newborn. Reiter's disease (urethritis, arthritis and conjunctivitis) was first described in 1918. The working definition is an episode of peripheral arthritis of more than 1 month's duration occurring in association with urethritis or cervicitis. There is a male:female ratio of between 10:1 and 50:1. Keratoderma blenorrhagica involving the soles of the feet and palms of the hands affects about 10% of patients. Treatment affects the urethritis but not the arthritis, which responds to non-steroidal antirheumatic drugs. Acute attacks resolve but recurrence affects up to three quarters of patients, about 10% being unable to work.

Herpes genitalis

Herpes simplex infections of the genitalia are on the increase. In 1976 7500 new cases were reported in Britain but in 1980 there were 10 800 – about 2% of all diagnosis. It is an acute infection characterized by small groups of blisters on a reddened base and a tendency to recur.

There are two types of herpes virus. Type 1 is usually found in lesions of the face, lips, mouth and tongue and type 2 is found more frequently in the genital area. This distinction is not entirely clear-cut but the virus can be demonstrated under the electron microscope and grown inside fertile hen eggs.

Symptoms and signs

An urgent symptom, especially in women, is the acute onset of pain, although the eruption may be preceded by some discomfort and itching. The eruption is vesicular and individual lesions are arranged in several groups. Erosion of the vesicles occurs leading to the development of superficial ulcers which can run together to form larger erosions in skin or mucous membrane. Crusting occurs and healing is usually complete in 7–14 days, but there is often painful enlargement of inguinal lymph nodes.

In men lesions occur on the penis, prepuce or glans and in women on the vulva, perineum, urethral and periurethral area, vaginal introitus and cervix. Primary attacks are usually more distressing than recurrent attacks, especially in women who may have a severe systemic illness requiring hospital admission. Micturition may well be extremely painful and acute retention of urine can occur.

If the cervix is the only area involved the lesions are unlikely to be noticed, and the presenting feature is then pelvic pain due to iliac and para-lymph node involvement.

Secondary infection can occur, resulting in deeper ulceration, tissue destruction and delayed healing.

Diagnosis

The clinical diagnosis is typical but it can be confirmed by trans-
ferring material from the ulcers onto a swab stick and placing this
in virus transport medium. Inoculation onto tissue culture
material in the virus laboratory will be followed by a cytopathic
effect within 48 hours. Dark ground illumination of serum from
the lesion can also be employed.

Management

Unfortunately, two well-publicized features of herpes genitalis remain true. It is a recurrent disease and no cure has been discovered. Palliative remedies should be employed, however. Normal saline applied locally will help to prevent infection and
encourage healing. Local application of idoxuridine and other antiviral agents has proved disappointing and as they are expensive
they should not be used. Local anaesthetic oitments may help but
there is an ever-present and real risk of hypersensitivity.

Systemically, analgesics are very likely to be necessary and in
the presence of secondary infection co-trimoxazole two tablets
b.i.d. will promote healing.

Acyclovir for intravenous, oral and topical use was introduced
in 1982 and is an antiviral agent which does appear to reduce the
duration of viral shedding, healing time and the duration of symptoms in patients with primary herpes and in recurrences; it is the
first of a new generation of antiviral agents which appear safe for
systemic and topical use. Unfortunately, it does not prevent recurrences. Tablets are much less effective than i.v. administration.
Herpes vaccines have been developed but none have been tested
in double blind trials.

Complications

Recurrences are common in men and women but they are usually
less severe and painful than the primary attack. Although the
majority of patients have recurrent attacks, only a few have
attacks occurring every 3–4 weeks which significantly disturb the
patient's sexual life. The factors which provoke recurrence are not
understood but sexual intercourse is often implicated.

Herpetic lesions in pregnancy can be dangerous as the virus may cross the placenta into the fetal circulation, producing disseminated intravascular coagulation and fetal death. Lesions involving the birth canal at the time of delivery may produce encephalitis, keratoconjunctivitis, hepatitis or cutaneous herpes in the child. Elective caesarian section is often carried out. However, up to 70% of babies with neonatal herpes are born to mothers with no symptoms or signs. There has been thought to be a link between herpes simplex virus 2 and cervical neoplasia. The exact role, however, remains to be verified and the relationship is not fully established or proved. However, cytological examinations should be carried out annually in women who have acquired the virus.

Genital warts

Genital warts usually occur in crops on the external genitalia of men and women. They have a viral aetiology and the incubation period may be many months. Perianal warts are not unusual, especially in homosexual men, but autoinoculation and spread by hand is common. Condylomata acuminata is an alternative name for the lesions, which are pinky-brown raised areas with a tendency to form a cauliflower-shaped mass.

Treatment can pose problems because of a tendency to recur. First and foremost scrupulous cleanliness is mandatory. Soap and water twice daily followed by careful drying should be followed by painting the lesions with a solution of 10% or 25% podophyllin in alcohol on alternate days, taking care not to involve healthy flesh. When the warts are hard, glacial trichloracetic acid will be required in minute quantities applied carefully with a cotton stick or fine swab. Widespread masses may require cauterization or curettage under local or general anaesthesia. Scissor excision is a new technique and involves injecting normal saline into the subcutaneous tissues. The ballooning of the tissue causes the warts to stand proud and they are snipped off from the skin with surgical scissors. Healing is usually rapid and pain minimal. There is increasing evidence of a link between genital warts and cervical cancer. Frequent cervical smears are recommended.

Syphilis

Syphilis is declining in incidence. The number of new cases of syphilis seen at clinics increased during the 1970s to a peak of 4866 in 1978. However, in 1946 the postwar peak was five times greater at 27 761. The 1980 figure was 4460. Annual deaths from syphilis in Britain declined from 213 to 101 between 1968 and 1978. The condition is commoner in homosexual men, over half the cases resulting from homosexual contact. It is divided into three stages. The primary stage is characterized by an ulcer at the site of infection, the secondary stage by generalized lesions on skin and mucous membrane and the tertiary stage, which occurs much later, by gummatous and destructive lesions.

The organism

Treponema pallidum is a corkscrew-shaped organism with a bluish-white appearance when seen in the dark ground illumination of a microscope. Sexual intercourse is the usual mode of transmission and the organism must be present on the skin or mucous membranes. The incubation period varies from 9 to 90 days with an average of 25 days.

Symptoms and signs

Primary syphilis. The primary chancre begins as a small raised papule, round or oval in shape, which develops into an ulcer with an indurated and well defined border. It is usually painless, as are the associated regional lymph glands which have a rubbery consistency. Without treatment, healing takes place in 3-8 weeks. In men, common sites are the coronal sulcus, the glans penis, the prepuce near the fraenum, the external urinary meatus and in homosexual men the anal margin. Women develop chancres on the labia, the fourchette, the cervix, the urethral orifice and the clitoris. Extragenital chancres are found on the lip, tongue, tonsils and nipples.

Secondary syphilis. During the secondary stages which develop 6-8 weeks after the primary, 80% of patients have skin lesions usually involving palms and soles or lesions of the mucocutaneous junctions, 50% have generalized enlargement of the lymph nodes, 30% have lesions of the mucous membranes and 10% involvement of the meninges, the uveal tract of the eye or liver and spleen. Symptoms are variable and mild; malaise, fever, headache and sore throat are usually common. The secondary lesions are extremely infectious, as is the primary chancre.

Tertiary syphilis. Tertiary syphilis may develop 2–20 years after initial contact, after a latent period during which serological tests are positive. The most typical lesion is the gummatous ulcer which may involve skin, subcutaneous tissue, mucous membrane and bone. However, viscera, the cardiovascular system and the nervous system may also be involved, a classical feature being the neuropathic joint.

Diagnosis

The diagnosis of primary syphilis is bacteriological. *T. pallidum* is found in the serum from the chancre, using dark ground illumination. At this stage serological tests are of limited value. The diagnoses of secondary syphilis and tertiary syphilis are helped by serological tests. Tests include the Wasserman reaction (WR) – a complement fixation test; the Venereal Disease Research Laboratory test – a flocculation test; Fluorescent Treponemal Antibody test; treponemal immobilization test; and the *Treponema pallidum* Haemaglutination Assay. Remember that previous exposure to yaws and certain collagen vascular diseases and glandular fever can cause a positive WR.

Treatment

Penicillin is the treatment of choice. Procaine penicillin 600 000 units i.m. daily for 10 days is usually recommended. Tetracycline or erythromycin 500 mg 6-hourly for 15 days is an alternative approach in allergic patients but the regimen should be repeated after 3 months. The prognosis of treated early syphilis is good, with a failure rate of under 15%. Biological cure, the complete eradication of treponema from the body, occurs in 80-90% of patients. No patient with persistent positive serological tests for syphilis should be discharged from follow-up.

Latent syphilis is treated by penicillin as in early syphilis. Late syphilis is also treated by penicillin but preliminary prednisolone is advised to reduce the incidence of the Jarisch-Herxheimer reaction.

Congenital syphilis

Congenital syphilis is really a prenatal infection transmitted by the mother to the child through the placenta. Clinical manifestations include the early infectious syphilis signs, the late non-infectious manifestations occurring after the second year of life and the stigmata (Hutchinson's teeth, nerve deafness and interstitial keratitis).

THE ROLE OF THE GENERAL PRACTITIONER IN THE SEXUALLY TRANSMITTED DISEASES

The general practitioner is responsible for the primary and continuing care of a defined population of patients who have registered with him for that very purpose. In contrast, the service for sexually transmitted diseases in United Kingdom was set up as a result of the Venereal Disease Regulations passed by Parliament in 1916. A confidential service was required and all 230 NHS clinics offer free access with or without a letter from the general practitioner who will only be advised of the patient's attendance and treatment if he refers the patient or the patient specifically requests it. Indeed, only four patients were included as having new episodes of venereal disease in 1982 in DB's practice and all were first diagnosed there.

Despite the fact that the general practitioner will be unaware of the fact of treatment in the vast majority of his patients with serious disease, he still has a crucial role to play in disease prevention, health promotion and the management of established disease and its effect on patient and family.

Treating the sexually transmitted diseases

Despite the existence of the clinics, the general practitioner will still treat many diseases, often without referral. Very few patients with trichomoniasis, molluscum contagiosum, genital warts, candidosis, tinea cruris, scabies or pediculosis pubis will be referred to specialists in genito-urinary medicine. The general practitioner may well wish to manage many women and men with herpes virus infections and a few patients with gonorrhoea when they present initially to him, especially if the idea of a clinic attendance should be distressing to them. Adler (1982) points out that there is no reason why general practitioners should not do their own micro-biological and serological investigations but they *must* be prepared to make an accurate microbiological diagnosis using tests performed from the correct site and they *must* ensure that sexual contacts are seen.

Disease prevention and health promotion

Sexually transmitted diseases are preventable diseases. The general practitioner's main strength lies in the personal relationship he has developed with his patients which has been founded on the successful past management of health problems whether new, continuing or recurrent. This relationship, however, should not be idealistic, starry eyed or naive. If it is, the patient will not wish to disturb it by bringing up sexual problems. The general practitioner must always be prepared to discuss sexual behaviour and sexual problems openly and frankly when the situation requires it and often by bringing up the subject first. There are groups of patients particularly at risk. Patients with marital difficulties are an at-risk group as are those whose work takes them away from home. Opportunities for health education will arise during many first consultations for contraceptive advice, particularly when the patient is young and unmarried or unattached. Many men who attend with minor blemishes on the penis are quietly terrified of venereal infection and they should be given an opportunity to express their knowledge about infection so that it can be updated by the general practitioner. The use of the condom has been shown to offer significant protection during casual sexual contacts.

Finally, more general practitioners are becoming involved with health education in schools and health education via the media, whether writing or appearing on radio and television; sexually transmitted diseases are important topics to cover.

Screening

The study carried out by Adler and colleagues (1981) suggests that wide-scale screening for gonorrhoea in women is not justified in general practice. This study was supported by Hiscock (1982) who carried out an 18-month study in a general practice with 8000 patients. He found no gonorrhoea in an asymptomatic group of 338 women, trichomonas in 6%, candidosis in 14%, warts in 2% and herpes in two patients. As far as symptomatic women were concerned, however, 3% of 173 women had gonorrhoea, 13% tri-chomonas, 37% candida, nine women had herpes and eight had warts.

Thirty-eight men presented with symptoms. One had syphilis, five had gonorrhoea, 11 had non-specific urethritis, 11 candida, 11 warts and one herpes. These figures emphasize the need for proper bacteriological diagnosis in general practice.

The psychological and social problems

Personal and interpersonal problems not only lead to the acquisition of a sexually transmitted disease – they also develop from them. The skilfully introduced statement about the temptation to stray when marital difficulties crop up in consultations, coupled with statements about the risks of sexual infection, may well provoke therapeutic discussion. Many patients who have acquired sexually transmitted diseases benefit greatly from the opportunity to discuss their problems with their general practitioner, particularly if they feel themselves to be the innocent victim. Occasionally the general practitioner is asked by a spouse for advice on how to introduce the subject to a partner, particularly a wife when she has unknowingly been exposed to the risk of infection. The authors believe that the contact is no less a patient than the victim and has a right to the truth if she deliberately seeks it. There can be no justification for deliberately lying about the need for investigation and treatment, and the reason for it, when sexually transmitted disease is suspected or discovered; after all, complications may follow. However, the reasons for investigation of a vaginal infection, including swabs and smear test, are often complex and discussions can reveal just as much (and no more) than the patient seems to want to know. A statement that the spouse might have the same problem as the wife or husband may avoid much marital disharmony. Having said all this, however, it is still surprising how often the revelation that a patient has gonorrhoea is followed by an apparent lack of interest in how precisely the infection was acquired. A patient also has the right not to know.

Contact tracing

By far the best method of tracing contacts (which is essential if sexually transmitted diseases are to be controlled) is to ask the patient to list sexual partners and inform them that treatment may be required. If people do not attend, they can be followed-up. Married men are often reluctant to name their wives and some contacts may be so brief that names are not exchanged.

In 77% of clinics, contact tracing is carried out by designated non-medical personnel, many of whom have had no formal training. Practice Health Visitors could help in this work if necessary. All should read the *Handbook on Contact Tracing in Sexually Transmitted Diseases* published by the Health Education Council.

REFERENCES AND FURTHER READING

Adler, M. W., Belsey, E. M. and Rogers, J. J. (1981). Sexually transmitted diseases in a defined population of women. *Br. Med. J.*, **283**, 29

Adler, M. W. (1982). The G.P. and the specialist – genito urinary medicine. *Br. Med. J.*, **284**, 1677

Adler, M. W. (1982). Contact tracing. (Editorial) *Br. Med. J.*, **284**, 1211

Adler, M. and Mindel, A. (1983). Genital herpes hype or hope. (Editorial) *Br. Med. J.* **286**, 1767

Catterall, R. D. (1979). *Venereology and Genito Urinary Medicine*. 2nd Edn. (London: Hodder & Stoughton)
Hiscock, E. (1982). Sexually transmitted diseases in a general practice. *J. R. Coll. Gen. Practit.*, **32,** 627

8

Gastrointestinal Infections

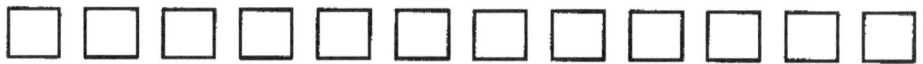

INTRODUCTION

Gastrointestinal infections are a very important cause of morbidity in the United Kingdom and a very important cause of morbidity worldwide. The incidence of specific gastrointestinal infections is rising, even in Britain in the 1980s, but investigation and subsequent notification of a patient with a gastrointestinal infection occurs in only a small proportion of patients presenting to the general practitioner. Diarrhoea may be the major work of the few large infectious diseases units in the United Kingdom, but many of the people who suffer from the increasingly recognizable infections do not even contact their general practitioner, let alone end up in hospital. The identifying of the patients who should be investigated and the even harder selection of those who need hospital admission will be mentioned specifically with each infection. Isolation of the patient from family and friends is seldom justified, providing personal hygiene is good, but if the physical condition or social circumstances of the patient merit hospital admission, isolation facilities should be sought, particularly if profuse diarrhoea is the problem. Vomit is seldom infectious.

TREATMENT (GENERAL)

The mainstay of treatment of gastrointestinal infections, however severe, is the maintenance of fluid balance with the replacement of lost body fluid. A small percentage of sugar (2–4%) of either glucose or dextrose in the replacement fluid, when taken by mouth, helps in the absorption of the salt and water. With the right solution, it is even possible to replace all the fluid lost orally. This applies even in a case of severe cholera.

SYMPTOMATIC TREATMENT

Antiemetic and antidiarrhoeal agents are seldom justified and undoubtedly overprescribed. In many cases they could even be harmful.

Acute infantile gastroenteritis

Viral infections (particularly rotavirus) account for the majority of cases of acute infantile gastroenteritis. Several large surveys of children admitted to hospital indicate that 75% are 6 months to 1 year and the condition is much commoner in bottle-fed babies[1]. Rotavirus occasionally occurs in adults. (The oldest rotavirus infection seen by EMD in 1983 was in a 77-year-old female who needed intravenous fluid replacement.)

Causes

Main causes are:

Rotavirus
Adenovirus
Noawalk agent
Calicivirus
Astrovirus

Other causes of infantile gastroenteritis are numerically less important than rotavirus but all the pathogens seen in adults are, of course, capable of causing gastroenteritis in children:

Campylobacter
Salmonella

Toxigenic *E. coli*
Shigella
Clostridium difficile toxin
Giardia lamblia
Cryptosporidium
Amoebic dysentery

Antiemetics

Antiemetics are occasionally justified in the treatment of vomiting associated with gastrointestinal infections but are much more useful when dietary indiscretion is the cause of the upset. Most agents have some sedative properties, particularly the antihistamine compounds.

Metoclopramide intramuscularly can sometimes allow rehydration to continue orally but should only be used when the cause of the vomiting is reasonably obvious.

The mainstay of oral rehydration is small quantities often.

Antidiarrhoeals

A large number of antidiarrhoeal agents are available and even widely advertised in the lay press. None do anything to combat the infective process, not even the so-called antitoxins like kaolin and kaopectate.

Antidiarrhoeal agents should be used for what they are, social corks - useful for important occasions such as air flights but potentially very dangerous.

The anticholinergic drugs (particularly the atropine-and-diphenoxylate combination of Lomotil) can even cause respiratory depression in children, urinary retention (especially in elderly males) and blurring of vision. In many cases the drug, particularly Imodium (a preparation of loperamide hydrochloride), can exacerbate the colicky pains, one of the more unpleasant symptoms of gastroenteritis.

The diarrhoea itself could be the most important mechanism in the resolution of the infection and plugging the exit with a pharmaceutical cork too soon may well lengthen and worsen the course of the illness. Most patients when given this simple explanation will use antidiarrhoeals sparingly and sensibly.

The commonest mistake, particularly in elderly patients, is not stopping the antidiarrhoeal medication when the diarrhoea subsides (not necessarily stops). The inbuilt idea of 'finishing the course' can lead to severe constipation with a return of colicky abdominal pain and 'diarrhoea' – overflow being an important mechanical cause of diarrhoea.

Antibiotics

Antimicrobial chemotherapy is very seldom justified in the treatment of gastroenteritis in general practice. The indications are:

(1) Invasive salmonellosis (co-trimoxazole, amoxycillin, chloramphenicol) including the enteric fevers (typhoid, paratyphoid)

(2) Shigellosis (not *S. sonnei*) (the most common treatment used in the Regional Infectious Diseases Unit in Manchester being naladixic acid)

(3) Severe campylobacter infections (erythromycin)

(4) Severe yersinia and specific parasitic infections, particularly amoebic dysentery and giardiasis

Hospital admission or investigation should be seriously considered before antibiotics are used in the treatment of diarrhoea.

INVESTIGATION OF A PATIENT WITH DIARRHOEA

Very few patients who present with gastroenteritis to their general practitioners have stool specimens examined. Undoubtedly more should – but not many more, or the laboratories would be swamped in very short order.

It is very important to send specimens on *food handlers* and, unfortunately, this does not only mean waiters/waitresses or cooks. Barmaids, air hostesses and the housewife who does the school dinners twice a week should also be included. In an outbreak, a cook who is discovered to be excreting salmonella is often a victim and not the cause.

Patients living in institutions – local authority homes, boarding schools etc – should be considered for investigation. Very rarely is the first case in an outbreak investigated.

Anyone who has recently returned from abroad probably merits investigation (see Chapter 13).

Three stool specimens are not often sent, although this is the number recommended. A food handler normally has to have six consecutive negatives for salmonella but three are probably enough for shigella and campylobacter (campylobacter sometimes only two).

RETURN TO WORK

If a person is *fit* to start work, i.e. a cook excreting salmonella, but cannot do so for public health reasons, their general practitioner should sign them off as fit to work and the Medical Officer of Environmental Health will have to stop them working (an exclusion order) and it then becomes his/her responsibility to make up their normal wages (Public Health Act 1968). This is particularly important to part-time workers, i.e. less than 20 hours a week, who may receive virtually nothing if categorized only as being off sick. There is therefore considerable pressure on general practitioners from Community Physicians to keep people on sick pay.

TREATMENT OF INFANTILE GASTROENTERITIS

Parental education is the most important part of the treatment of infantile gastroenteritis. They should have explained carefully:

(1) Fluid replacement is the mainstay of treatment

(2) Antidiarrhoeals and antibiotics are contraindicated

(3) Hygiene is important, as the condition is infectious in most instances (hand washing and careful disposal of nappies the most important points)

Fluid replacement needs to be with a suitable solution in adequate volumes given at least initially by small quantities often[2]. Food withdrawal in the older child is a well-tried, time-honoured addition, but as yet has no scientific basis. Milk withdrawal, initially in younger children, followed by the gradual reintroduction through 25%, 50% and 75% strength feeds over 36 hours is also time-honoured, with no control studies as yet.

What solution?[3]

Currently available preparations readily dilutable are convenient but relatively expensive.

It is very important to mention specifically that high solute solutions, particularly the well-advertised strong sugar solutions, are contraindicated. The use of isotonic fluid feeds has helped to reduce hypernatraemic dehydration dramatically but, particularly in older children, the reasonable demands of an ill child for something nice to drink should not be paramount.

Table 8.1 Composition of the commonly available oral preparations for maintaining fluid balance in diarrhoea (in mmol per litre)

	Dioralyte	Rehidrat	WHO fluid
Sodium	35	50	90
Potassium	20	20	20
Chloride	37	50	80
Bicarbonate	18	20	30
Glucose	200	91	111
Sucrose	—	94	—

The WHO fluid is now made up using plastic spoons with a large end for sugar and a small end for salt. It produces very variable quantities of sodium chloride and sugar, depending upon the quantities used.

Amount given

Maintenance fluid is $2\frac{1}{2}$ oz/lb (150 ml/kg), per day and should be increased to 3 oz/lb (200 ml/kg) (minimum) when fluid loss continues.

Commercial preparations

The two most often used are:

(1) Dioralyte: this has now been reintroduced without colouring (cherry brand had been withdrawn because it looked like blood in the stools)

(2) Rehidrat (lemon and lime)

A simple solution of a teaspoonful of sugar and a pinch of salt in a pint of water does well in the emergency situation.

How much fluid to recommend is the most difficult thing for a general practitioner to calculate or estimate. It is perhaps the one occasion when that terrible Americanism, guesstimate, is justified.

(1) If there are obvious signs of dehydration, e.g. sunken eyes, sunken fontanelle, loss of elasticity of the skin etc, hospital admission is justified. If the child is quiet and listless, a 'blue light' admission is justified. If 15% or more dehydrated the mortality is 50%.

(2) The fatter the child, the more difficult it is to detect dehydration.

(3) Maintenance fluid orally is 5 ml/kg per hour approximately. To this quantity should be *added* an estimate of recent losses (5% of actual weight).

(4) It is very difficult to be precise about the child's weight. Recent clinic weights would be useful but very few mothers are actually aware of a recent weight. The weight can be taken as the 50th centile for the child's age, remembering that some adjustment can be made for parental size. As long as rehydration is oral, overestimation is safe provided it is in small quantities often, to avoid vomiting. To this end, fluid is best prescribed, at least initially, in ml per hour. If there are difficulties over ml and – incredibly – only fluid ounce measures available, the fluid intake should be 3 oz/lb per day.

Re-visit

Very few children, however small, will need a re-visit providing clear instructions are given at the first. The clearest instruction, however, should be not to hesitate to call again. Infantile gastro-enteritis is probably the commonest condition where the situation changes dramatically in less than 24 hours - fortunately, almost always for the better.

Parents should be warned to look for persistent vomiting (oral rehydration ineffective). The diagnosis would need to be reviewed. The infant should continue to pass urine although the diarrhoea would subside. Dry nappies (three or four in succession) should merit at least another telephone call if not another visit.

GENERAL DISEASE PATTERNS

Much more is now known about gastrointestinal infections and the mechanisms by which they produce disease but epidemiologically there are two main ways.

(1)   By multiplication of organisms outside the patient and production of toxin which when ingested makes the patient ill a short time after ingestion (classical staphylococcal food poisoning at 2-4 hours after ingestion)

(2)   By ingestion of organisms which then multiply inside the gastrointestinal tract and produce the illness. The common infections of campylobacter and salmonella produce an illness in this way. The viral gastroenteritis of childhood and even the less common infections of the Coxsackie and ECHO viruses can also be inhaled as well as eaten.

The organisms which multiply inside the gastrointestinal tract can also produce two basic clinical pictures, although a great deal of overlap is common. Rotavirus infection produces an enteritis where the small bowel is predominately affected and large quantities of fluid can be lost. Shigella infection on the other hand produces more of a 'colitis'; although there may be frequent bowel actions they are small in quantity and tend to contain blood and mucus.

The latter presentation is more easily clinically confused with inflammatory bowel disease and the cardinal rule for general practitioners to remember is that infective diarrhoea very seldom lasts for more than *10 days*. Should a patient's diarrhoea become chronic, hospital referral to exclude inflammatory bowel disease should be considered even if a pathogen such as campylobacter has been isolated. Attacks of inflammatory bowel disease (Crohn's or ulcerative colitis) can be precipitated by an intercurrent infection.

Salmonella infections

Salmonella gastroenteritis has been overtaken by campylobacter infections as the commonest cause of gastroenteritis (Figure 8.1).

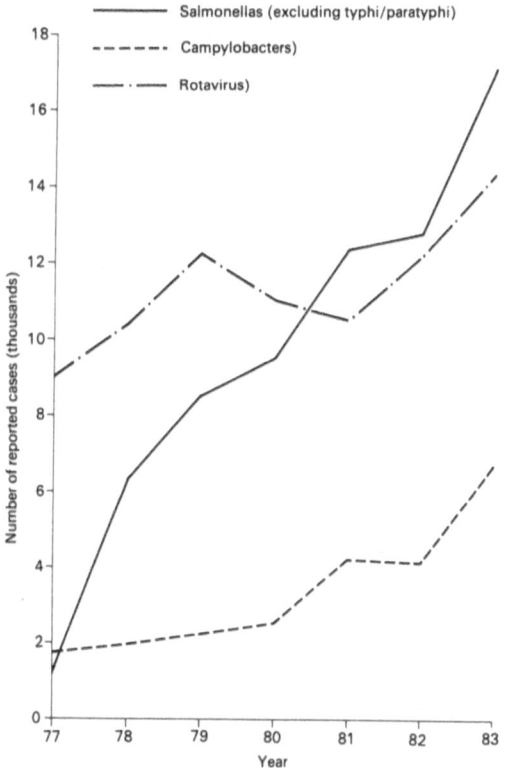

Figure 8.1   Graph showing gastrointestinal trends[4]

The reported incidence is still, however, approximately 20 per 100 000 population per annum and shows no sign of decreasing (remember notifications are a lot less than actual infections).

Salmonella are widespread in the animal world and almost all raw meat in the United Kingdom, particularly poultry and beef, produced with intensive methods will contain salmonella. Deep freezing doesn't kill them but proper cooking does. The commonest mistake is to thaw incompletely before cooking, but proper storage (refrigeration) of cooked meat and the cleaning of surfaces and utensils that have been contaminated by the raw meat or blood are the most important precautions.

Faecal-oral spread is a less common, but important, factor and infected food handlers should be excluded from work.

Clinical illness

The clinical illness is typically an acute gastroenteritis with colicky abdominal pain and vomiting as well as diarrhoea. The fluid loss can be alarming (enteritis) but blood and mucus in the stool are not uncommon. The incubation period is usually at least 12 hours, but can be 48 hours – so blaming the immediately preceding meal is not correct in most instances. 'What did you eat yesterday or the day before?' or 'when did you last eat out or have a "take-away"?' are more appropriate questions.

Treatment

Antibiotics should not be used except in very severe cases and where bacteraemia is suspected. In most cases where antimicrobial chemotherapy is considered, hospital admission is necessary. The very young and the elderly are particularly susceptible and any patient who has had gastric surgery (even 40 years ago) is much more at risk. It is not just a question of stomach acid killing bacteria, as patients on cimetidine and other H_2 antagonists do not seem to carry the same risk.

Excretors

The commonest problem encountered by most general practitioners is the chronic excretor. About 5% of patients affected excrete the organism in their faeces for 3 months or more. Again the very young and the elderly are inclined to be longer secretors. Even then treatment is seldom justified and patients with known gallbladder disease can theoretically be 'cured' with long courses of antibiotics (2 months of co-trimoxazole or amoxicillin). Chloramphenicol is probably the best drug for acute severe life-threatening salmonella infections but its use on carriers cannot be justified.

The general practitioner should not sign 'well' carriers off sick but leave work/nursery/school exclusion to the Medical Officer for Environmental Health (see Return to Work, page 123).

To facilitate regular specimen collection and also to alter the colonic pH (more acid) a small dose of lactulose (Duphalac) – not enough to cause diarrhoea – is sometimes justified.

Figure 8.2 gives an example of types of salmonella likely to be found.

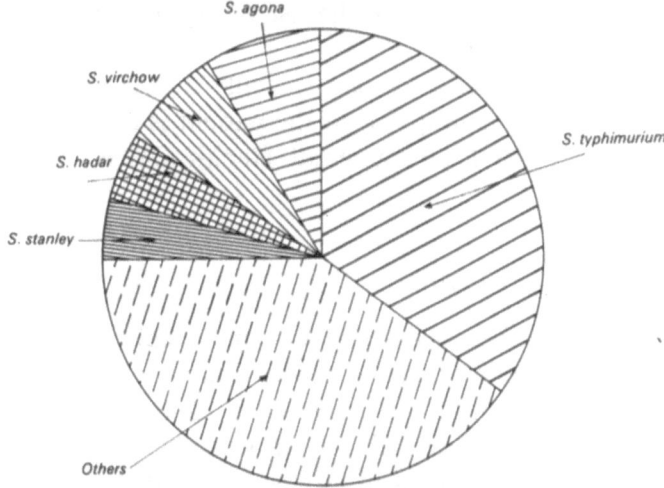

Figure 8.2 Pie chart to illustrate the main types of salmonella isolated at the Regional Infectious Diseases Unit, Manchester

Campylobacter infections

This relatively recently described cause of gastrointestinal tract infection has become the commonest recognized infection in adults (see Figure 8.1). The laboratory conditions necessary for its identification are exacting and probably account for its anonymity until recently. There are a number of different species and stereotypes and most are widespread in nature. The commonest source to man is poultry, and undercooked chicken is often the cause of an outbreak of food poisoning. Puppies with diarrhoea are another cause of infection transmitted to man and several large outbreaks have occurred with contaminated milk.

Campylobacter food poisoning has a reasonably long incubation period, 3–5 days, and is noted for severe abdominal pain and blood in the faeces although neither is universal. Intussusception is often suspected in infants and appendicitis in adults. The mainstay of treatment is fluid replacement and spontaneous recovery the rule. Erythromycin is often used, as the organisms are sensitive; several double blind trials have shown very little improvement over placebo, however, but the worst is often over before diagnosis is made (48 hours to isolate the organism is a rule). If a rapid test becomes available the use of erythromycin may have to be investigated again.

Campylobacter enteritis is *not* officially notifiable (except perhaps under food poisoning) but if the patient is a food handler or hospital worker the Environmental Health Officer ought to be notified.

Clostridium difficile toxin

An increasing number of cases of *C. difficile* colitis caused by the production of a toxin from the bowel organism are being recognized in the community. In a year-long survey at the Regional Infectious Diseases Unit (RIDU) it was the third commonest cause of infective diarrhoea in adults admitted directly from the community (see Table 8.2).

Table 8.2 Isolations in RIDU study

Campylobacter spp.	58
Salmonella	46
C. difficile toxin	14
Shigella flexneri	5
Shigella sonnei	3
Other shigella	2
Plesiomonas shigelloides	2
Aeromonas	1
Vibrio parahaemolyticus	1
E. histolytica	2
Giardia lamblia	2
Total	136

Monsall Hospital Adult Diarrhoea Study

A total number of 412 patients were admitted with acute diarrhoea and in approximately one third an infective cause was found. Constipation with overflow was common and other causes included diverticulitis, carcinomas and inflammatory bowel disease.

Pseudomonas colitis

Pseudomonas colitis (the severe end of the spectrum of difficile colitis) was first described in surgical units following powerful broad spectrum antibiotics like clindamycin. The commonest cause of difficile colitis in the survey was amoxicillin. Remember that the diarrhoea problem often starts *after* the antibiotic course has been completed.

Treatment with metronidazole and vancomycin by mouth is effective but relapses are not infrequent. Vancomycin is much more expensive but in the Regional Infectious Diseases Unit has been found to be marginally more effective.

Shigella dysentery

Shigella dysentery is usually an unpleasant, acute diarrhoeal illness with small, frequent stools containing blood and mucus. It has a mean incubation period of 48 hours and can be very unpleasant.

Shigella sonnei is currently the commonest in the United Kingdom and is fortunately the mildest type. Sonnei rarely needs, or gets, specific treatment. *S. flexneri*, *S. shigae* and *S. boydii* are usually treated because antibiotic treatment has been shown to improve symptoms and decrease excretion. Unlike treatment of salmonella there is no increase in carriage rate.

The family practitioner is most likely to come across the problem with a child kept off school because he/she is still excreting shigella. Unless the child is quite old (over 8 years) and has impeccable hygiene this is a wise precaution. However, most children will have acquired the infection from the school toilets in the first place. Shigellas are more infective than most other bowel pathogens and can easily be caught from 'dirty' toilets, door handles and towels.

A week's treatment with nalidixic acid (Negram), 250–500 mg four times daily, can be useful in many cases of prolonged absence but should not be used in every case.

Cryptospiridiosis

In the past 2 years another infection causing gastroenteritis in both adults and children has become readily identifiable by many laboratories. The protozoan cryptospiridia has been associated with the family and community outbreaks of diarrhoea and vomiting[1]. It is identified by microscopy of faeces stained with a variation/modification on Ziehl–Neelsen direct smears staining and sputum for acid-fast bacilli.

Cryptospiridium is similar to *Toxoplasma gondii* and is most vicious in immunocompromised patients (in whom it may never get better) but the diarrhoeal illness can last 2 weeks in 'normal' individuals. Treatment is relatively ineffective, the best of ineffective treatments probably being the macrocide antibiotics – spiromycin.

The illness tends to be more of an enteritis with fluid loss, although a colitic type is not unknown. In the immunocompromised a malabsorption state is well recognized.

Spontaneous recovery is the rule and, as with many other self-limiting gastrointestinal infections, most cases will not even be specifically identified.

WORM INFESTATIONS

Threadworm

The only common worm infestation in Britain is the threadworm (*Enterolius vermicularis*). In some studies as many as 20% of the population studied had threadworms. The only real problem to the patient is perianal itching, particularly at night when the eggs are deposited. The gravid females are sometimes seen perianally, and in faeces as tiny cotton-thread-like organisms only a few millimetres long, but the best method of diagnosis is using a cellophane (e.g. Scotch) tape applied perianally, in the early morning, and then examined for the eggs. If the diagnosis is in doubt a general practitioner should easily be able to arrange for a Scotch tape to be applied and then stuck on a glass slide which could then be sent to the local laboratory for examination. This is seldom necessary.

Treatment

General practitioners should explain that although personal hygiene is important in eradicating the infestation, that doesn't mean that poor personal hygiene was the cause. Most children acquire the infestation in school and bring it home.

Piperazine, 2 g daily for 7 days, is usually effective – but remember that *all* the household should be treated at the same time. The drug does not kill the worms but loosens their hold on the colonic mucosa and purgation is essential if the alternative single 4 g dose is used.

The *house* should be cleaned, especially the toilets, and the bed linen laundered to remove the eggs.

The commonest causes of treatment failure are chronic constipation and reinfection from unremoved eggs.

Mebendazole (Vermox) is actually cidal to the worms and is a good alternative but cannot be given to very young children (under 2 years). The usual dose is 100 mg (one tablet) per week but 100 mg daily for 6 weeks is very effective and very safe. Much larger doses have been used for echinococcus infections.

Other worms

The general practitioner occasionally encounters other infestations but they are very rare and usually in patients who have been infected abroad.

Human roundworms (Ascaris lumbricoides)

Ascaris is passed *per rectum* or coughed up. It conforms most closely to what lay people think of as a worm and is usually more unpleasant than actually symptomatic. Occasionally very heavy infestations can cause intestinal obstruction or bile duct obstruction but the commonest complication during migration is a significant eosinophilia and an allergic reaction.

Treatment. Piperazine is the treatment of choice as a single dose of 4 g for adults.

Tapeworm

Tapeworm infestation is usually brought to the patient's attention when he or she asymptomatically pass in the faeces a segment (it looks like uncooked flat ravioli). Do not handle the segment, as pork tapeworm can be directly infectious through the skin. Treatment is usually effective with niclosamide and purgatives but it is no longer necessary to look for the 'head' segment, as niclosamide causes disintegration. Pork and beef tapeworm are caught from eating undercooked meat, the other tapeworm, which is very rare but has caused a lot of controversy recently, is *Toxocara canis* (dog tapeworm) with reported incidence of congenital eye infections.

Rarest infestations

There are many other rare worm infestations that a general practitioner may come across. The clue to invasive parasitaemia will be an eosinophilia and should not be ignored. A general practitioner sent a young man from the Cameroons to see a psychiatrist because he complained of worms crawling across his eyes. A short course of diethylcarbamazine (Banocide) was curative for his *Loa loa*. Banocide should always be taken at first under medical supervision as unpleasant anaphylactoid reactions can occur.

There are several useful serological tests for worm infestations and amongst those used by EMD regularly are hydatid, schistosoma and filarial.

Many weak positive results, however, may not need treatment and expert advice about diagnosis and treatment of infestations is usually justified as they are all rare and there have been many improvements in therapy in recent years. Praziquantel (a single oral dose treatment for schistosomiasis) is a case in point but EMD treats less than a third of the cases referred.

Hydatid cyst

Occasionally an elderly patient is discovered to have a hydatid cyst. It is best left alone as surgery is usually more hazardous than the disease and if surgery is indicated in a young patient with local symptoms it is best done in specialist referral centres.

REFERENCES

1. Ellis, M. E., Watson, B., Mandal, B. K., Dunbar, E. M. and Mokashi, A. (1984). Contemporary gastro-enteritis of infancy: clinical features and prehospital management. *Br. Med. J.*, **288**, 521-3
2. Ellis, M. E., Pope, J. and Benjamin, S. (1981). Management of gastro-enteritis at home. *Br. Med. J.*, **283**, 1606
3. Cutting, W. A. M. and Ellerbrock, T. V. (1981). Homemade oral solutions for diarrhoea. *Lancet*, **1**, 998
4. Communicable Diseases Report, Weekly Edition, 84/01

9

Hepatitis; AIDS

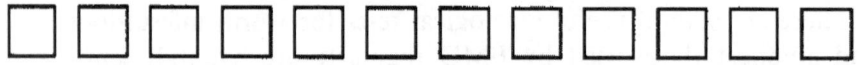

INTRODUCTION

Hepatitis is an acute viral infection which is remarkably 'organ' specific. Although most patients who have been diagnosed in the past will tell you that they have had 'yellow jaundice', most people affected by the commonest virus do not become jaundiced. Estimates vary between 1:10 and 1:30 with the majority of adults joining the ubiquitous 'flu-like' illnesses and most children going 'off their food' for a few days, or more, rarely a few weeks. There are three main categories:

(1) Hepatitis A (formerly infectious hepatitis)

(2) Hepatitis B (formerly serum or Australian antigen hepatitis)

(3) Hepatitis Non-A, Non-B

The third category is the rarest and is only diagnosed by excluding (1) and (2) on serological tests. It is probably at least two viruses (almost certainly more than two), one of which is transmitted like hepatitis A (faecal–oral) and one transmitted like hepatitis B (parenterally).

Numerous other viruses cause hepatitis as part of their protein manifestations – most notably Epstein–Barr (glandular fever), where as many as 80% of clinically-affected cases will have raised transaminases and 20% may even be clinically jaundiced. Cytomegalovirus can cause a predominately hepatic clinical picture. Herpes simplex, enteroviruses, rubella and influenza can all cause a hepatitis, usually in addition to their normal effects.

SIZE OF THE PROBLEM

For the first half of 1982 notifications of infective jaundice in England and Wales were between 1000 and 1200 every 4 weeks, representing a fivefold increase since 1980. The increase was, in the main, accounted for by hepatitis A, as laboratory reports of hepatitis B positive tests remained constant at just over 200 per 4-week period.

Despite the fact that hepatitis A is endemic throughout the world and some population developing countries can have serological evidence of 97%, the UK General Practitioner will only see a clinical recognizable case of hepatitis A every 2-3 years and will only see two to three cases of serum hepatitis throughout his entire career.

Hepatitis A does occur in sporadic outbreaks and a local colleague in a small group practice confirmed 20 cases on the same housing estate over an 8-week period. Only one required hospital admission (for social reasons) and two were seen in Outpatients for prolonged convalescence (no further treatment was recommended).

Hepatitis B is more common in many parts of the world than in Britain. In England and Wales the carrier rate in healthy blood donors is less than 0.1%. In Greece and other areas of eastern Europe, this rises to between 5% and 10% and in some parts of West Africa and south-east Asia it can be as high as 20%. One of the cases seen in recent years by EMD was a young woman who had a spontaneous abortion whilst on holiday in Egypt and was given two units of blood.

It is estimated by the WHO that there are 200 million carriers of hepatitis B worldwide.

INCUBATION PERIODS

Hepatitis A is usually transmitted by the faecal-oral route and has an incubation period with a mean of 28 days (6 days-6 weeks).

Hepatitis B is transmitted parenterally or sexually and extremely rarely by conjunctival splash. Mothers who are known to be positive frequently transmit the virus to their offspring in the postnatal period. Its incubation period is much longer than hepatitis A and probably depends to some extent on the number of virus particles involved in the exposure. On average the incubation period is approximately 100 days with a variation of 1–6 months.

DIAGNOSIS

The history of an insidious onset over 2–3 days with lethargy, anorexia, nausea and right upper quadrant pain after exercise or eating should suggest the diagnosis of hepatitis and often the urine becomes very dark before jaundice develops.

Arthralgia and rashes make the diagnosis more likely to be hepatitis B.

A history of contact with person or persons who have recently had jaundice is very common.

Even in the United Kingdom hepatitis is a disease of the younger ages and, unless a definite solid contact history is available, the diagnosis is suspect in anyone over 30 years of age, when the major differential diagnoses become more common.

DIFFERENTIAL DIAGNOSES

Biliary tract disease or excess alcohol consumption can mimic viral hepatitis and both can cause pancreatitis, which can mimic severe hepatitis in its own right. Autoimmune hepatitis, drug induced jaundice (with or without hepatitis) and carcinoma (usually secondary or pancreatic) can all present like viral hepatitis.

Agents which cause jaundice/hepatitis

These commonly include:

(1) alcohol

(2) phenothiazines (chlorpromazine)

(3) anaesthetics (halothane)

(4) antituberculous drugs (rifampicin, isoniazid, pyrazinamide)

(5) methyldopa

(6) contraceptive pills

(7) organic solvents (e.g. carbon tetrachloride) - not forgetting the increasingly notorious 'glue', sniffed or otherwise

If the patient has recently returned from abroad yellow fever, the most virulent of all types of viral hepatitis, must be considered. The patient may have malaria or even an amoebic liver abscess. The three main causes of viral hepatitis are all more common in areas where malaria and yellow fever are found than they are in the United Kingdom.

If yellow fever, malaria or amoebic liver abscess are suspected, urgent hospital admission should be sought.

Cholangitis secondary to biliary obstruction should be suspected when the patient is toxic, has swinging temperature and a good story for rigors. Haemolytic anaemia can present with jaundice but the symptoms of anaemia - i.e. tiredness and malaise - should be distinguishable from the tiredness and malaise of the 'flu-like' prodrome of hepatitis.

Gilbert's disease

Every general practitioner should be aware of the existence of Gilbert's disease. It is usually discovered by accident when a patient who is just vaguely unwell, possibly with a minor viral infection, is thought to be jaundiced.

The liver function tests usually confirm the fact that the bilirubin is slightly raised but the rest of the liver function tests are normal. This finding may recur on several occasions when the patient is just vaguely unwell.

Its only clinical significance is that it should be recognized. It is an inherited condition of delay in bilirubin transport and further investigations should be avoided if at all possible as it usually involves invasive manoeuvres, such as liver biopsy. In practice the best way to avoid investigation of an otherwise well patient is to avoid specialized referral.

Leptospirosis

Leptospirosis is a rare but well-recognized differential of hepatitis. Most doctors remember the risk to sewer workers, but of the approximately 60 cases per year in Britain, most work in contact with animals on farms, the dairy industry in particular. Leptospirosis is a disease of workingmen, slaughtermen, sewer repair men (much more likely to be cut) and also is associated with certain hobbies, freshwater fishermen and people who like swimming in canals especially.

Clinical features to suggest leptospirosis include:

(1) sudden onset,

(2) severe myalgia,

(3) oliguria and conjunctival haemorrhage,

(4) meningism or frank meningitis.

(5) neutrophil leukocytosis (in viral hepatitis there is usually a mild leukopenia).

The liver bilirubin is markedly raised with barely abnormal transaminases (usually 1000+ in hepatitis, in leptospirosis 100–200 at the most). If there is a relevant history (occupation or exposure), penicillin should be given whilst awaiting laboratory results. After the onset of the immune complex phenomena of renal failure and severe haemorrhage, giving penicillin probably makes very little difference. Survival usually depends upon good intensive care with dialysis.

Little can be done to prevent occasional massive fatal haemorrhage. Only two or three patients die in Britain annually but the reported incidence of 60 cases per year is an underdiagnosis, as many patients will have a self-limiting 'flu-like' illness without a trace of jaundice and do not even contact their general practitioner, never mind end up in hospital.

INVESTIGATIONS

When taking blood from suspected hepatitis cases remember the following.

(1) Wear gloves. (Nobody does all the time - but see below, the patients most likely to have hepatitis B)

(2) Do not stick the needle in either yourself or the nurse, and dispose of it wisely. (Don't replace in plastic guard - drop it straight into the container)

(3) Ensure, as far as possible, that not a drop is spilt

(4) Label all specimens 'high risk' and send them to the laboratory in *separate* plastic bags with the relevant forms. All blood should be taken into screw-topped plastic bottles. (Put in *separate* plastic bags so that any leakage of one specimen won't ruin the other samples)

Liver function tests

Transaminases should be at least ten to 20 times the normal but 100 times is not uncommon. The level of transaminase is *not* an indication of the severity of the hepatitis. Gamma GT (more elevated than SGOT, SGPT) may help to differentiate alcohol or drug induced hepatitis.

Hepatitis B surface antigen test should be sent to the nearest laboratory, usually the local PHL or regional laboratory service. Most local DGHs will have a forwarding service.

Urine for bilirubin/urobilinogen is worthwhile, particularly if neoplastic obstruction is suspected, where urobilingogen can be totally absent.

In cases of viral hepatitis, the white blood count is usually low or normal.

The transaminases are usually markedly elevated at 3000–4000, which is commonplace, but the actual rise is *not* significant prognostically. Also remember that in many young people (especially around puberty) the alkaline phosphatase is much higher, due to growing bones. A high alkaline phosphatase with only moderate transaminase rise is suggestive of an obstructive jaundice.

Some patients are more likely to have hepatitis B than hepatitis A. Intravenous drug addicts and male homosexuals are particularly at risk. Close contacts, especially sexual contacts, of known cases or carriers are at risk, as are residential staff of mental hospitals, subnormality schools and custodial institutions, particularly overcrowded closed prisons.

Approximately 2% of the working population work for the National Health Service and some of them are also at special risk (special risk being defined as greater than the general population). The groups of National Health Service workers at an increased risk of hepatitis B used to be those associated with renal dialysis units. Indeed, two outbreaks, one in the Manchester area in 1965/66 and one in Edinburgh in 1969/71, caused the deaths of several NHS employees. The current practice of screening staff and patients has greatly reduced the risk. There remains, however, an increased risk above the general population for many groups of NHS workers, particularly casualty officers or those working in the blood transfusion service or people working in units with a special interest in hepatitis (either Infectious Disease Units or Gastroenterological Units) and those who also work with drug addicts.

The most important test prognostically is the prothrombin time (also the most often forgotten). Any patient with a prothrombin time of 20 seconds (normally 12–13 s) one should consider for hospital admission. Greater than 30 seconds, hospital admission is strongly advised, and greater than 40 s+, fulminant hepatic failure is a distinct possibility and hospital admission is mandatory. Special bottles are necessary for the estimation of prothrombin time and should be kept in the *fridge*; they are usually 2.5 ml, and are generally available from the local district general hospital.

MANAGEMENT

Most patients with hepatitis A can be nursed at home. Symptomatic relief of the nausea, abdominal pain and vomiting can be obtained with bed rest and a low-fat diet taken in frequent small amounts. There is no evidence, however, that even the strictest bed rest or diet speeds recovery. Most patients should be symptomatically improved in 2-3 days and physically recovered in 2-3 weeks.

Alcohol should be voided completely, for 6 months, as should the contraceptive pill. No other medication should be taken if at all possible. Some patients obtain relief from 'indigestion' with small doses of alkali; mist. magnesium trisilicate is probably the best, as aluminium salts would increase the likelihood of constipation. Cholestatic phase towards the end of the illness can produce intense itching and symptomatic relief can be obtained with oily calamine or crotamiton 10% cream (Eurax). A prolonged cholestatic phase, where simple remedies fail to produce relief, should reopen the possibility of obstructive jaundice. The initial febrile illness obviously present could have been due to cholangitis.

A simple non-invasive investigation of abdominal ultrasound is fairly reliable in excluding extrahepatic obstruction of the bile ducts. This investigation should be available after consultation, with your local radiologist, on an outpatient basis.

Hospital admission

Most hospital admissions for hepatitis are for social reasons, particularly the lack of support in the home environment. However, there are a number of important medical reasons to look out for.

(1) Drowsiness; any decrease in the level of consciousness and falling off of higher mental functions (not just tiredness)

(2) Any overt bleeding or a particularly prolonged prothrombin time. In certain circumstances it might be best to repeat the test before requesting hospital admission i.e. a very well patient clinically not agreeing with the test

(3) Inadequate fluid intake, particularly the development of ketosis

143

(4) Slow resolution, particularly in the development of the cholestatic phase

Remember above the age of 30, the older the patient the less likely
is their jaundice to be due to hepatitis.

RETURN TO WORK

The commonest decision a general practitioner has to make about
a patient who has had hepatitis is when they should go back to
work or school. In practice it has nothing to do with infectivity
but depends on the patient's well-being and the physical demands
and nature of the work. There are some people, e.g. surgeons and
theatre nurses, who should not go back to work whilst they remain
hepatitis B positive.

The two authors cannot agree how long a consultant physician
or general practitioner should stay off work after hepatitis A, but
both would suggest that a psychiatrist could go back to work in
less than 2 weeks!

COMPLICATIONS OF HEPATITIS

Fulminant hepatatic failure leading to death despite modern intensive care still occurs and is probably numerically more common
with hepatitis A. It is, however, incredibly rare. Long term complications following hepatitis A are non-existent. In the acute
phase death is due to cerebral oedema or more rarely severe
haemorrhage.

Hepatitis B and Non-A, Non-B can of course lead to fulminant
hepatic failure in their own right. Long term complications of
hepatitis B depend upon 'e' status. If the patient is unlucky enough
to be one of the very few patients who remain 'e' antigen positive
and 'e' antibody negative they have a chance of developing cirrhosis and/or hepatoma.

INVESTIGATION OF A CARRIER

Occasionally the Blood Transfusion Service refuses to accept
somebody as a blood donor because hepatitis B surface antigen

was found on screening. Under normal circumstances, the patient's general practitioner is informed by letter and hospital referral recommended. The general practitioner is not obliged to refer providing that he or she:

(1) Confirms the test result by repeating it

(2) Examines the patient for any signs of chronic liver disease (spider naevi, leukonychia, liver palms, hepatomegaly or splenomegaly)

(3) Checks the liver function tests (these are usually normal, emembering that the screening test could be positive in the 'incubation' period of the llness)

(4) In the event of the positive test being confirmed, arranges for 'e' status to be examined. Whether the patient is 'e' positive (and remains so) will determine his or her infectivity and likelihood of complications. Chronic active hepatitis, cirrhosis, liver failure and even hepatic carcinoma are all more likely if the patient is 'e' positive; 'e' positively is taken to mean the continuing replication of virus

(5) Counsels the patient on what the above results mean. Changing the lifestyle, indulging in sexual intercourse and attitudes to simple everyday occurrences such as nose-bleeds are important. However, it is also very important that the patient does not go away feeling like a leper and that he is a danger to his friends and family. It is particularly important to warn him about future hospital admissions, operations and dental work, where his attendants should be made aware of his status

The delicate balance between adequate warning and not frightening the patient into a hermit existence is one which is not easy to strike. Treat 'e' negative as non-infectious except for donating blood and surgical (including dental) procedures.

IMMUNIZATIONS

Normal human gammaglobulin can be used to prevent hepatitis A. The efficacy wanes from a few days after the intramuscular injection until, several months later, no protective effect is left. 750 mg (× 3 amp) will last approximately 6 months but only 250 mg (1 amp) is all that is necessary in most cases.

Gammaglobulin is most commonly used for overseas trips (see Chapter 13) but is occasionally indicated in the United Kingdom when a close contact of a recently diagnosed case is pregnant or immune suppressed. It is *not* indicated in an outbreak in an institution, e.g. school. The best preventive measures are hygienic. Disposable towels, cleaner toilets and more frequent handwashing are far more effective.

Hepatitis B vaccine (Morsen)

Hepatitis B vaccine is offered to health care workers at special risk and household contacts of hepatitis 'e' positive patients. This is given by three intramuscular injections over a 6-month period – the first two injections 1 month apart, and the third 6 months later. Originally it was in very short supply but because of the scare about AIDS it has not been taken up – the scare arose because the vaccine was manufactured from the blood of New York homosexuals. Treatment of the vaccine to render it safe is in three stages (immersion in 8 mol/litre urea; the pepsin at pH2 and formaldehyde). Any one stage is viricidal. Its manufacture is completely different to other blood products like Factor VIII for haemophiliacs which would be destroyed, along with the virus, if so vigorously treated.

What evidence there is available suggests that hepatitis B vaccine may be protective against AIDS. Of 1800 practising homosexuals who have been vaccinated, three have developed AIDS. In 3000 controls, 56 have developed AIDS. This may just reflect more social responsibility in the vaccinated group, of course.

AIDS

AIDS stands for the acquired immune deficiency syndrome. The aetiological agent is a retro-virus, human T cell lymphotropic virus type III (HTLV-III).

AIDS has generated great anxiety in the United Kingdom fuelled by some unnecessary sensationalism of the mass media, particularly the less reputable national press.

The main reasons for anxiety are that it is a new disease with no known cure and an unpleasant downhill course. The number of cases in Britain is increasing and up to the end of 1984 there were 118 cases with a steady increase predicted. The disease is extremely serious for the individuals affected but it is *not* highly infectious. In the UK only practising homosexual males (over 90% of cases) and patients such as haemophiliacs who receive large amounts of blood products have been affected. In the USA and Europe intravenous drug abusers have been affected as well, but *not* to any extent in the UK.

The general practitioner when presented with a patient who might have AIDS can deal with the patient himself in the first instance if he/she wishes. HTLV-III antibody testing is available and a reasonably reliable screen is an ordinary white blood count and differential where an absolute lymphocyte count over 2000 would make AIDS very unlikely.

Clinical clues to AIDS include recent weight loss, persistent lymphadenopathy, unexplained florid Candida or herpes simplex.

In the future the general practitioner is much more likely to have a patient who is HTLV-III positive but who is perfectly well. If the patient is homosexual he should be encouraged to change his lifestyle in terms of steady partners, non-penetrating sexual activities and encouraged to consult one of the advisory services available (e.g. Terrence Higgins Trust, BM AIDS, London WC1N 3XX. Tel: 01-278 8745).

The incubation period is as yet unknown but is probably at least two years, and if the patient develops lymphadenopathy, becomes short of breath or develops any odd skin lesions urgent hospital referral is necessary. The other major presenting complaint is persisting diarrhoea lasting more than ten days.

The two commonest problems in AIDS patients are Kaposi's sarcoma and *Pneumocystis carinii* pneumonia. Kaposi's sarcoma is a deep-seated dark purple lesion of the skin often found peripheral but can occur anywhere. *Pneumocystis carinii* pneumonia is very amenable to treatment (high dose co-trimoxazole or pentamidine) but should be diagnosed before the chest X-ray is abnormal if possible. The GP should tell any patient who is HTLV-III positive (man or woman) not to have children because of the very high risk of congenital AIDS.

147

10

Central Nervous System Infections

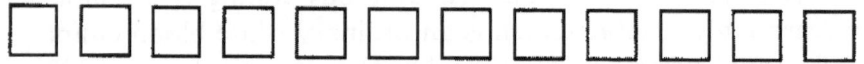

One of the rarest but potentially most serious of all infections encountered by the general practitioner is an infection involving the central nervous system (c.n.s.). Meningitis and encephalitis are two distinct entities; although an element of both is usually present, one predominates, and they are usually discussed separately in most medical textbooks. To the average family doctor meningitis, or suspicion of meningitis, is an easier diagnosis to reach because of its cardinal signs. Encephalitis, however, merges into the differential diagnosis of toxic confusional states, epilepsy, drug overdose and major psychiatric illnesses. Encephalitis is also occasionally included in the differential diagnosis of cerebral vascular accident (CVA) especially if the patient is febrile.

ENCEPHALITIS

Encephalitis can be broadly classified into two categories:

(1) acute brain destruction

(2) post-infectious encephalitis

Acute brain-destroying encephalitis

This is typified by herpes simplex when the organism multiplies inside the brain substance and behaves like, and is indeed a type of, cerebral abscess (usually multiple). The patient usually presents with febrile illness and focal neurological signs, with or without grand mal convulsions. In the older patient the diagnostic trap is the much commoner cerebral vascular accident – always be suspicious when a CVA has any history of recent febrile illness or indeed is febrile when first seen.

Post-infectious encephalitis

Almost every infection (particularly viral) has been recorded as a possible cause of post-infectious encephalitis. Although it is much commoner than the more vicious tissue-destroying invasive encephalitis – Type 1 (approximately four times as common) – the average general practitioner will only see one or two cases in his whole career.

The childhood exanthemata of measles and chickenpox plus the orthomyxo (influenza) viruses are the commonest cause. In the USA mumps is classified as the single most common cause, but the distinction between mumps meningitis and mumps encephalitis is not often made the other side of the Atlantic – hence the keenness on mumps vaccine in the United States.

Size of the problem

The incidence of herpes simplex encephalitis is probably somewhere between one and two cases per million population per year. The United Kingdom would therefore expect to have between 50 and 100 cases per year, with a total number of cases of all encephalitis being approximately five to ten times that figure (herpes simplex varies between 10 and 20% as causes of encephalitis). There is, however, probably an underestimate, with very mild cases going undiagnosed.

General practitioners should suspect encephalitis following a febrile illness when personality changes and headache are accompanied by a decreased level of consciousness. Focal signs are usually absent and convulsions less common than many think. Post-chickenpox encephalitis is almost always a cerebellar encephalitis and the adult, or more usually the child, will usually appear drunk and suffer motion sickness. The uncoordinated movements will be much easier to detect when the patient is not in bed, a good pointer to the fact that bed rest is advantageous, and the use of drinks with straws (so that the patient doesn't have to move the head) can sometimes maintain oral hydration.

Treatment

Hospital treatment is probably necessary for all but the mildest cases. Hospital treatment is necessary to consider the question of herpes simplex, but the commonest reason is probably the nursing care of the semiconscious patient. A cmbination of depressed consciousness and vomiting can lead to the disaster of aspirated vomit - probably the commonest cause of death in the milder post-infectious type.

Recovery and return to normal activities

Post-infectious encephalitis completely returns to normal, usually within 3 months. However, minor degrees of neurological deficit can persist.

With invasive types (typified by herpes simplex), permanent damage is usual but recovery can go on up to 18 months to 2 years after the illness. Until recently it carried a *mortality of* 70% but 33% is now more common with intensive care and antiviral agents[1,2].

MENINGITIS

Inflmmation of the meninges surrounding the brain has several causes other than infections. Chemical (usually following myelograms) and carcinomatous or leukaemic invasions are amongst the others, but general practitioners will see acute infections. Viral infection will be the commonest cause but bacterial meningitis (approximately 1200 cases per year in the UK) is much more serious and still carries a high mortality (5-50% depending on types). Any first-year clinical student should be able to diagnose meningitis in a patient with an acute illness, high fever, vomiting, severe headache, marked neck stiffness and unbearable photophobia. However, not all the cardinal signs will be present in most cases and yet again the very young and the elderly are the ones most at risk. In the case of meningitis the very young have a cardinal sign of their own, the bulging fontanelle, but a continually screaming infant often appears to have a bulging fontanelle. The quiet, listless infant with a bulging fontanelle is the one with meningitis.

Viral meningitis is the commonest c.n.s. infection that general practitioners see. Between 1000 and 1500 cases are 'notified' in England and Wales per year. Many of the milder cases may well not be notified. Almost half the cases will be due to the ECHO viruses and this can be important as the echoviruses are the one group which regularly cause a skin rash (see below).

Bacterial meningitis is a severe life-threatening infection and is a diagnosis which should be considered in any acutely ill patient, especially if he or she has a fever. The common problems which present as possible bacterial meningitis are:

(1) tonsillitis,

(2) enlarged neck glands (from whatever cause),

(3) pneumonia.

The other major causes seen by general practitioners will be musculoskeletal with neck injuries. If the patient then has a minor viral infection or becomes febrile for whatever cause, meningitis may be suspected.

Viral meningitis

The three commonest causes are the enteroviruses (small RNA viruses), ECHO, Coxsackie and the paramyxovirus, mumps.

The enteroviruses may have a biphasic illness with a mild diarrhoeal illness preceding the meningitis and some of the echoviruses may produce skin rashes (see below). General practitioners should remember that most cases of polio virus infection do not produce anything other than a viral meningitis and if there is any reason to suspect it (i.e. recent travel abroad) specific investigations may be necessary and these would normally be carried out in hospital. The specimen most likely to produce diagnostic confirmation is not the cerebrospinal fluid (c.s.f.) but tissue culture of the faeces. Serology is very disappointing in enteroviral infections.

The enteroviruses are famous for causing other illnesses such as pericarditis and myositis but all other manifestations other than mild diarrhoea or meningitis are rare.

Mumps meningitis

Mumps meningitis usually accompanies other manifestations of the disease, particularly the commonest, parotitis, but occasionally no other signs are present. Complications are extremely rare but total unilateral deafness has been recorded.

Management at home

If a general practitioner is confident that the patient has *viral* meningitis, then management at home is possible. Treatment consists of standard nursing care with adequate analgesia frequently (aspirin is often sufficient) and maintenance of fluid balance. To this end, antiemetics like metoclopramide (Maxolon), prochlorperazine (Stemetil) are useful. Remember they can also be given by suppository if necessary. The patient will benefit most from being nursed in a quiet, darkened room.

Whether or not the patient can remain in his or her own home will depend on social circumstances but mostly on the confidence of the family practitioner that the patient does not have bacterial meningitis.

Bacterial meningitis (Figure 10.1)

The commonest bacteria to cause meningitis in the United Kingdom are meningococcus, *Haemophilus influenzae* and pneumococcus. The first two, meningococcus and haemophilus, are very much diseases of childhood with over half the cases of meningococcus being in the under-4-year-olds, and *H. influenzae* even more so, with half the cases being in the 1–4-year age group plus a third in the under-1-year-olds.

Pneumococcal meningitis, however, has 40% of its cases in the over-45-year age group – but still has over a third under 14 years of age.

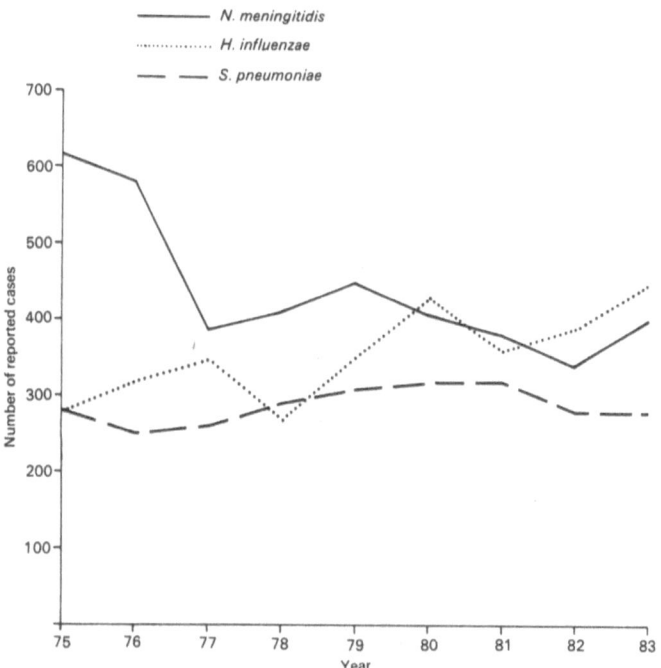

Figure 10.1 Graph showing incidence of bacterial meningitis

Management

The family practitioner's job is to make or suspect the diagnosis as soon as possible and request a blue light admission. If there is reason to suspect meningococcal meningitis by the presence of a purpuric rash (which may not be florid) or even if there is any purpura found at all, an injection of benzylpenicillin $\frac{1}{2}$-1 megaunit (300 000–600 000 u) intravenously if possible, but more likely intramuscular, should be given as soon as possible. Pay no attention to irate registrars complaining about difficulty in diagnosis if the blood or c.s.f. fails to grow the organism because of prior treatment. Better a live diagnostic problem than a dead diagnosis.

Bacterial meningitis in children usually has no preceding illness but occasionally a sore throat or ear infection has been diagnosed recently. Do not be worried if you have prescribed an antibiotic. It may have made the diagnosis more difficult but it may be the main reason why the patient survives undamaged.

The overall mortality of meningococcal meningitis is 5–10% and *H. influenzae* meningitis 3–6%, but pneumococcal meningitis has a mortality of 20% – which reflects not only the age of some of the patients but also the fact that it can follow skull or facial fractures, sinusitis and intracranial operations.

Prophylaxis

The family practitioner may be asked to prescribe prophylaxis for one of his patients who has been in close contact with a case of meningitis. Prophylaxis should be confined to close household contacts of the same age or younger. Prophylaxis for parents, grandparents, uncles and aunts is a waste of time but occasionally nursery groups or dormitory groups (boarding schools, scout camp etc) need prophylaxis. Until recently only contact with meningococcal meningitis required prophylactic treatment. There is some evidence that the practice should be extended to include *H. influenzae* cases but not pneumococcal ones.

Rifampicin at 10 mg/kg to a maximum of 600 mg as a single daily dose for 3 days is the treatment of choice. Swabbing the patient beforehand is not necessary because the very few secondary cases that occur are usualy negative but the positives, who would usually be carriers, may yield good epidemiological information.

Long term consequences

Most cases of bacterial meningitis recover completely but some are damaged, particularly if there has been a delay in diagnosis. A complete development assessment should be done 3–6 months later to detect any decrease in performance (hearing loss would be the commonest). Specialized help can minimize handicaps, however slight. Return to school or work is dependent on physical well-being (whether it was bacterial or viral meningitis) and long term problems are rare.

Recurrent headaches are not uncommon for some months and reassurance is usually all that is necessary. If the headache is accompanied by fever or any other symptoms like photophobia, then re-referral should be sought urgently, particularly if the initial problem was pneumococcal.

GUILLAIN–BARRÉ SYNDROME (post-infective polyradiculitis; polyneuritis)

Polyneuritis is a rare event which most general practitioners will see only once in their careers. It can follow virtually any infection, among the commonest being mycoplasma, glandular fever and influenza, but usually only a minor upper respiratory tract infection precedes the problem and an aetiological agent is proven in a minority of cases. In the Regional Infectious Diseases Unit in Manchester with full investigative facilities, in only 20% is the aetiology found.

The classical ascending paralysis is usually preceded by some sensory disturbance and the cardinal sign of loss of peripheral reflexes is important. The symptoms may be only minor but careful assessment is necessary on more than two visits if the general practitioner intends to keep the patient at home. It is particularly important NOT to prescribe sedatives or strong analgesia and urgent referral is necessary if any respiratory, coughing or swallowing impairment is suspected. It is particularly important to rule out poliomyelitis, even in the 1980s, but the major differential diagnosis would be multiple sclerosis and the older the patient the more likely would be a hidden malignancy.

A domiciliary visit is probably the best way of deciding if it is safe to keep the patient at home, but in all but classical cases hospital investigation is necessary, particularly as lumbar puncture must be included.

TOXINS AFFECTING THE NERVOUS SYSTEM

The classical toxin-produced infection is tetanus, fortunately now extremely rare. Others include botulism and various organic and inorganic poisons.

Tetanus

If a patient consults his doctor with difficulty in opening the mouth or with unusual muscle spasms, the diagnosis of tetanus should be entertained. A history of previous trauma recently is not always discovered. The commonest problem in the 1980s is dyskinesia due to medications like metoclopramide (Maxalon) or perphenazine (Fentazin) and in seven of the last ten cases referred to the Regional Infectious Diseases Unit in Manchester as tetanus, the cause has been a drug reaction. Immediate relief can be obtained by intravenous injection of Cogentin or Kemadrin.

Other causes mimicking tetanus would be dental problems, particularly molar or wisdom teeth, and temporomandibular joint problems or jaw dislocations.

REFERENCES

1. Whitley, R. J., Soong, S. J., Dobin, R. *et al.* (1977). Adenine arabinoside therapy of biopsy-proven herpes simplex encephalitis. *N. Engl. J. Med.*, **297**, 289–294
2. Sköldenberg, B., Forsgren, M., Alestig, K., *et al.* (1984). *Lancet*, 707–711

11

The Common Infectious Diseases

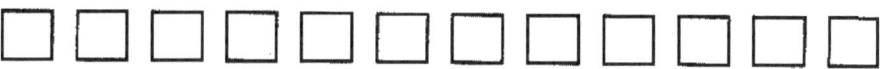

INTRODUCTION

Almost all the population of the United Kingdom will suffer from the common infectious diseases at some time in their lives unless successfully immunized against them.

Some of the infectious diseases, e.g. chickenpox, do not have an effective immunization and improvements on any large scale, particularly new immunizations, in this century are very unlikely. Even when an effective immunization is available, e.g. mumps, the balance of the morbidity and mortality of the disease versus the immunization programme and its complications may be such that it is not routinely used in the United Kingdom.

The vast majority of the patients seen by general practitioners with the common infectious diseases will be treated with simple symptomatic relief medication and suffer no complications whatsoever. In many instances it is not even necessary to isolate the patient, but historical practice in keeping a child off school until all the spots of chickenpox, for instance, have healed serves no useful purpose. Many of the diseases are far more infectious before the diagnosis can be made than afterwards. This is certainly the case in measles, mumps and whooping cough.

MEASLES

Measles is highly infectious and most children in the United Kingdom will suffer from it before they go to school (commonest incidence 2–5 years) unless they have been immunized against it.
Adult measles may become a problem in the future if immunization campaigns are only partially successful (see Chapter 2).
Measles has been considered part of 'growing up' for so long that
many people have lost sight of the fact that it is a very unpleasant,
miserable illness and still *kills* approximately 20 children every
year in the United Kingdom. Complications are, however, very
rare and even the commonest complication (otitis media) affects
only 2% of cases.

Diagnosis

The diagnosis of measles is relatively easily made once a few cases
have been seen, and most grandmothers are better at it than recent
medical graduates, who may not see a case until at least their
second or third postgraduate year. There are, however, a few basic
hints to avoid pitfalls.

Measles primarily affects the respiratory system and is very
similar to influenza except it produces a rash and a widespread
lymphadenopathy. The diagnosis should only be made if the child
has a substantial cough. The rash is an expression of the body's
response to the virus, and children with leukaemia or other unpleasant immuno-suppressive illnesses die from measles without
ever producing a rash. The rash can be very difficult to see on
black skins. The erythematous maculopapular rashes caused by
the semi-synthetic penicillins (ampicillin, amoxil) and by the sulphonamides are often described as morbelliform because they look
like measles. Last, but by no means least, measles under the age
of 9 months is very rare indeed (due to maternal antibodies).

Clinical course

The measles virus is inhaled and approximately 2 weeks later the
patient becomes ill with an unpleasant cough, conjunctivitis and

a high swinging fever. Some 3-5 days later a rash appears, usually behind the ears, and spreads down over the whole body, including the palms and soles, over the next 24-48 hours. The timing is important. All too often the young patient has been coughing and feverish and ampicillin or septrin was prescribed the day before the rash appeared. Widespread lymphadenopathy is in favour of measles. In this situation it is often difficult to be certain of the diagnosis. Koplik spots can sometimes be seen in the mouth before the rash develops but they are just the rash inside the mouth. The rash is erythematous maculopapular and coalesces a great deal before it fades leaving a brown 'measles' stain over the lighter skins. This stain is worrying to some mothers, particularly those of blonde girls, but they can be reassured that in time (occasionally months but usually a few weeks) it will fade completely.

Soon after the rash appears the temperature settles, and after a thoroughly miserable 4-5 days the child begins to feel better. If the temperature does not settle within a day or two after the rash appears look again for complications, particularly otitis media.

The respiratory rate should also settle but the detection of widespread crepitations in the lung fields does *not* mean secondary pneumonia has occurred as measles *per se* almost always causes 'crackles' to be heard.

Treatment

Simple antipyretic analgesia with aspirin or paracetamol plus occasionally some simple paediatric linctus for the cough is all that is needed. The miserable child usually feels better in bed but should *not* be confined to bed if he/she wants to be up and about. Variations in temperature are best avoided (i.e. the child should not be allowed out of the house).

Marked conjunctivitis which remains or becomes purulent is best treated with local toilet, and very occasionally an antibiotic eye ointment is necessary (i.e. chloramphenicol). The often marked coryza and perinasal crusting is best treated with soothing local applications, e.g. mother's cold cream or Vaseline, and *not* by frequent painful use of tissues. Bland oral fluids should be encouraged whilst the child is febrile.

Complications

Otitis media is best treated with amoxil/or some semi-synthetic penicillin as the organism most likely to cause problems in the pre-school child is *Haemophilus influenzae*.

Secondary bacterial pneumonia is also probably caused by *Haemophilus influenzae* but *Staphylococcus aureus* secondary infection is life-threatening and in most cases where it is suspected flucloxacillin should be used. Erythromycin in the first instance is a good substitute for both amoxil and flucloxacillin if the patient is sensitive to penicillin.

Very rare complications

These include sub-acute sclerosing panencephalitis (see Chapter 2). SSPE is incredibly rare and usually presents years after the initial infection. Epistaxis is occasionally the reason for measles cases to be admitted to hospital. Local treatment with packing is often sufficient but remember to *stop* the aspirin and substitute paracetamol if necessary. Appendicitis is an extremely rare complication of measles.

WHOOPING COUGH

The respiratory tract infection caused by the bacteria *Bordetella pertussis* is a very unpleasant, prolonged illness, particularly in the pre-school child, but can affect *all* age groups.

Whooping cough is probably becoming less serious and post-whooping cough bronchiectasis is almost unknown. It accounts for an average 12 deaths per year. Epidemics occur every 3–4 years in a population which is not immunized; most of the deaths occur in children under 6 months and most of the severe morbidity in the under-1-year-old children. The younger child has usually acquired the disease from an older sibling.

Clinical picture

The infection is acquired by droplet inhalation and 1–2 weeks later a nondescript upper respiratory tract infection begins with fever and coryza. At this catarrhal stage it is indistinguishable from hundreds of other respiratory tract infections and diagnosis is impossible on clinical grounds. During the second week the characteristic distressing paroxysmal cough begins and persists, particularly at night, for many weeks and sometimes months. The 'whoop' is the sudden drawing of breath at the end of the coughing and is often accompanied by vomiting. Even the worst case can look completely normal between attacks and therein lies the major diagnostic problem for general practitioners – a sudden distress call in the middle of surgery to find a perfectly well-looking infant on arrival. The history, not forgetting contact with a recent known case, is all-important. Many other respiratory illnesses, particularly para-influenza, adenovirus and respiratory syncytial virus, can mimic whooping cough but they are usually much shorter illnesses – 2 weeks as opposed to 2 months – and have no specific treatment of their own.

The rare diagnosis which is most important to bear in mind is the inhaled foreign body, and careful enquiries should be made at the first consultation.

The very young child (under 6 months) may not 'whoop' at all but just suffer from apnoeic attacks. These are, however, usually obviously ill enough to request urgent hospital admission.

Treatment

Antibiotics make little or no impact on the disease, although both erythromycin and cotrimoxazole make isolating the organism much more difficult and therefore presumably the patient less infectious. The use of erythromycin prophylactically is therefore scientifically sound but unproven, and should probably be given to both patient *and* younger sibling – 14 days being the usual course.

Good nursing is very important and because of the distress and vomiting the child should be fed small amounts often, but be disturbed as little as possible. Anti-tussive agents are best avoided.

VARICELLA ZOSTER

Varicella zoster is a highly infectious DNA virus that belongs to the herpes group. It infects almost everyone in the United Kingdom some time during their lives and causes two distinct illnesses:

(1) *Chickenpox*, with its vesicular rash which varies from six or eight spots confined to the thorax and upper abdomen to a widespread eruption which can cover almost all the skin.

(2) *Shingles*, which usually occurs later in life when immunity wanes, a recrudescence affecting one or two dermatomes unilaterally. Clinical observations suggest that if everyone lived to be 100 they would all suffer from shingles.

CHICKENPOX

Chickenpox has long been regarded as part of growing up, and is commonest amongst school children although it can affect any age group. Most cases are very mild and are easily missed, particularly if all the spots are under the vest. Several surveys of people entering medical school have shown that 85% have antibodies to V–Z virus but only approximately 50% will give a clear history of chickenpox.

The virus is shed in large numbers from the lesions on the skin and particularly from lesions inside the mouth. After inhalation by a non-immune subject, 13–17 days later the virus causes first a viraemia, then the rash develops in crops 2–3 days apart and taking 3–4 days to pass from vesicle–pustule–scab.

Most non-immune people in a single household will catch chickenpox from a single case. There is often no real prodrome although occasionally it may be 2 days before the vesicles are obvious. The patient remains infectious until all the scabs have healed, and traditionally is kept away from school or work until then. The general practitioner is often faced with a very healthy child with a few 'spots' remaining, who is not allowed back to school. The problem is most often with the teachers who worry about pregnant colleagues, etc., but if all the children acquired chickenpox in school then there would not be any non-immune teachers, and the incredibly small risk of congenital problems would disappear.

Treatment

Antipyretic analgesia is all that is needed for most cases, with a soothing lotion (e.g. oily calamine) to the skin. Itching and subsequent scratching can be a problem and oral antihistamines can help. Scarring, which is relatively rare, is much commoner when the lesions have been scratched with or without secondary infection.

Complications

The commonest complication is secondary skin infection and can be serious if widespread or not effectively treated. Antiseptic (such as Betadine paint) applied locally is usually all that is required, but any evidence of spreading cellulitis should be treated with oral antibiotics. *Staphylococcus aureus* is the main problem, and flucloxacillin or erythromycin for penicillin-sensitive patients are the first line treatments (see Chapter 12).

Neurological complications

Encephalitis is usually a cerebellar type with ataxia and slurring of speech. It is a transient demyelinating type (see Chapter 10), and total recovery is normal although hospital admission may be required for fluid balance and nursing care. A very rare complication is transverse myelitis which usually presents with back pain and retention of urine followed rapidly by weakness in the legs. Urgent hospital admission is mandatory.

Pneumonitis

A primary chickenpox pneumonitis is a very rare but very important complication. It occurs most often in young adults and occasionally kills. Any patient who develops an unpleasant cough or shortness of breath in the throes of chickenpox should be admitted to hospital urgently. Intravenous acyclovir (hopefully given before chest X-ray signs appear), and modern intensive care with artificial ventilation, dramatically reduces mortality. There will be no clinical signs apart from moderate to severe chickenpox lesions on the skin.

SHINGLES

The dermatomes most commonly affected are thoracic but the second commonest, the ophthalmic division of the trigeminal, causes the most problems. Paraesthesia and pain usually precede the vesicular eruption and the pain is often bad enough to mimic myocardial infarction or renal colic.

Treatment

Vigorous treatment of the zoster rash reduces the incidence of neuralgia but post-hepatic neuralgia is really only numerically important in patients *over* 50 years of age and many clinical trials which have not confined themselves to the older age groups have effectively been conducted on much smaller numbers than reported. 5% IDU (idoxuridine) in DMSO (dimethyl sulphoxide) is effective but 40% IDU in DMSO is more so. Until recently 5% IDU in DMSO (Herpid) was the only treatment readily available to general practitioners, but commercially 35% IDU has become available. Dimethyl sulphoxide is a potent antiseptic as well as a solvent (transports IDU through skin), and probably accounts for some of the effectiveness. It has a peculiar garlicy-onion smell which cannot be sensed by a significant minority of patients. Application of any preparation with DMSO is not recommended for longer than 4 days as it causes chemical burning of the skin, but can occasionally produce intolerable discomfort on the first application. 40% IDU is very expensive, approximately £1/ml, and for economical reasons is usually applied once a day with an occlusive dressing and the same dressing has a top-up addition of the fluid applied daily. Acyclovir cream (5%) may prove effective but a licence for the treatment of zoster has not yet been approved, although it is effective against herpes simplex (see p. 180).

Treatment of pain

The pain of shingles really occurs in two parts:

(1)   acute pain during the initial attack,

(2)   post-hepatic neuralgia.

(1) can merge into (2), which is generally much more difficult to treat.

Treatment of the acute pain

This will need rapidly elevating doses of analgesia – morphine and morphine derivatives are often required. The simple analgesia of aspirin and paracetamol is never sufficient in the over-50s but combinations of paracetamol and dextroprophoxyphene are sometimes sufficient. Temgesic, a sublingual application, has become a recent favourite. As an adjunct to all effective analgesia adequate night sedation (benzodiazepam) and aperients (lactulose or dorbanex) should be given to counteract the constipation of adequate analgesia. Waiting for the pain to break through before the next dose of analgesia is wrong, and frequent doses over the first week, and sometimes 2 weeks, are essential.

The dips in blood drug levels should not drop to the pain threshold if therapy is to be fully effective. Sometimes prednisolone as an anti-inflammatory agent is beneficial at this stage.

Post-hepatic neuralgia

This is far more difficult to treat than the ordinary pain of acute injury. The peculiar paraesthesia and lightning pains are difficult but no analgesia is adequate *alone*. The morphine derivatives are contraindicated because of addiction, but many additions can have some advantages:

(a)   amantadine,

(b)   carbamazepine (particularly useful with paraesthesia),

(c) locally applied analgesic creams and even mechanical (battery-operated) vibrators have their advocates.

Often nerve block with local anaesthetic is very beneficial. Use the short-acting lignocaine in the first instance and once the most effective spots have been found the long-acting marcaine (with adrenaline) can be effective for many days and even weeks after one injection. Remember to continue to use the other adjuncts of therapy – night sedation, aperients and even antidepressants.

Post-hepatic neuralgia can last for years in rare instances, and is usually associated with severe skin scarring; if all the above treatments are used skilfully, however, the patient will be able to lead a reasonable existence. Eventually permanent nerve block is very occasionally needed and specialist referral to pain clinics may be necessary.

Ophthalmic shingles

The first division of the trigeminal is the second most common dermatome affected. The skin area should be treated as other skin areas with shingles but the difficulty lies with the eye itself. Intensive treatment is often necessary to prevent scarring of the cornea and subsequent loss of vision. If the nasociliary branch is involved the eye will be affected and the clue for the general practitioner is to look closely at the *nose*. If the rash of shingles extends down the nose then the eye will be affected. Start eye treatment immediately – 3% acyclovir eye ointment or 2% idoxuridine (kerocid) two or three times a day. Steroid eye ointment often in combination with an antibiotic, e.g. Predsol-N (with neomycin), or the antibiotic can be given separately, e.g. chloramphenicol ointment. The pupil often needs dilating but remember the hazards of narrow-angle glaucoma in the elderly. All in-patients with EMD have slit-lamp examinations in ophthalmology out-patients, but if this is not practical then the author suggests that the general practitioner should treat vigorously as above.

NOTIFICATIONS

Notifications are regarded by many as an inaccurate record of what goes on, and of little importance. Most infectious diseases which are supposedly notified are not actually reported. The recent increase in fee (effective from August 1983) from 25p to £1.15 (the 15p is supposed to cover the postage) may lead to better reporting and an artificial increase in some infectious diseases.

When trends can be checked it is surprising how accurate the graphs can be. In influenza and whooping cough epidemics the large rise and fall of the notifications is 'mirrored' by a similar rise and fall in laboratory isolations (although with very much smaller numbers).

Notifications alert community physicians and environmental health officers to the possibility of outbreaks and local epidemiological problems. They are important in the general gathering of information and help in the assessment of vaccination programmes and the recording of complications, particularly as complication rates for most infectious diseases are very low. The only diseases which are commonly reported by general practitioners are: measles; whooping cough and food poisoning.

More rarely reported are: acute encephalitis, acute meningitis, dysentery, infective jaundice, malaria, enteric fevers (typhoid and paratyphoid), and tuberculosis.

The majority of notifiable diseases – acute poliomyelitis, anthrax, cholera, diphtheria, Lassa fever, leprosy, leptospirosis, Marburg disease, rabies, relapsing fever, scarlet fever, smallpox, tetanus, typhus fever, viral haemorrhagic fever, yellow fever and plague – are very rarely reported by anyone, never mind general practitioners. The general practitioner who reports more than one of the above diseases in his clinical lifetime is a rarity.

RUBELLA (German measles)

The rubella virus belongs to the family of Toga viruses, and except for congenital infection causes no serious illness. Rarely the complication of arthritis can cause problems. It usually affects the hands and fingers, and therefore mimics rheumatoid arthritis. However, the arthritis resolves completely usually within 2 weeks and has no sequelae.

Clinical features

There are no diagnostic parameters which are typical of rubella. Even occipital lymph node enlargement has no clinical significance and many people will acquire natural infection without developing a rash at all. Typically, however, the rash is like measles on the first day (without the prodrome and coryza). The patient may, however, have a cough and conjunctivitis. On the second day it becomes confluent and can look like scarlet fever (bright pink but not raised like the streptococcal infections) and on the third day it disappears.

The major differential diagnoses are the entero viruses (Echo and Coxsackie) and glandular fever (see pp. 170-4) but atypical measles and any minor infection complicated by a rash (drug or food allergy) should be included.

Management

The general practitioner's major problem with rubella is the patient who is known to be, or might possibly be, pregnant coming into contact with a suspected case.

The general practitioner needs to confirm the diagnosis of rubella. Confirmation and duration of pregnancy are also very important. The likelihood of congenital malformation is 90% if rubella is contracted during the first 10 weeks, 33% if contacted at 11-12 weeks and 19% at 13-16 weeks. Deafness, the commonest defect, occurs up to 20 weeks gestation.

Confirmation of diagnosis

The virus may be isolated from the throat by throat swab or nasopharyngeal aspirate. This simple investigation is most often forgotten and is even useful in the index case which is most often a small child (from the same family) on whom blood tests could be difficult.

The best method of confirming the diagnosis is by serology, looking for antibodies. The presence of antibodies may indicate past infection and a rise in titre (usually 4 times) or IgM antibodies is necessary. The first titre may be negative (also indicates no immunity) and a second sera 10–14 days later is essential. The patient need have *no* symptomatic illness whatsoever, but may still have been infected. Early consultation with the local virus laboratory is recommended.

In the early 1970s there were approximately 1000 rubella-related therapeutic abortions. In the early 1980s this has dropped to approximately 200 per annum. The incidence of congenital rubella cases has also dropped from an average of 67 cases (1970–75) per year to approximately 20.

If the patient is unwilling to consider termination then hyper-immune gamma globulin specific against rubella can be given. It should be given as soon as possible after exposure; its value is as yet non-proven but even if it only prolongs the incubation period it could be very valuable. Specific hyperimmune gamma globulin should normally be available from the local public health laboratory.

MUMPS

The mumps virus is an RNA virus which belongs to the paramyxo group and is first cousin to influenza and measles. It infects most people in their lifetime but of the recognized childhood illnesses it is probably the one which is most often remembered as affecting adults. This probably reflects the fact that it is less infectious than measles or chickenpox although, in some studies, 90% of adults have antibodies and at least 30% of cases are subclinical. Mumps is most often seen in the 5–15 age group and is generally a febrile nuisance more than a life-threatening disease. It is, however, prob-ably the single most common cause of aseptic meningitis taking the entero-viruses as separate entities (see Chapter 10).

Clinical picture

After inhaling the virus, some 18–20 days later the patient will develop fever and headache and even pain in the parotid before the characteristic parotid swelling develops 2–3 days later. In 25% of patients the parotid swelling is unilateral, and when bilateral can occur sequentially.

All the well-known complications of mumps can occur without the characteristic glandular swelling. Orchitis occurs in 20% of postpubertal males who catch mumps, and meningitis is more common in males than females.

Management

Antipyretic analgesia is all that is required in most cases. It is worth remembering that bland food and drink do not stimulate the salivary glands as much as 'tasty' do. The commonest reason that a general practitioner treats mumps is orchitis, although females can develop oophoritis, which is often missed.

Orchitis

Most often this is unilateral, and pain develops before swelling. An athletic support (jock-strap) is well worth using, and if aspirin or paracetamol do not produce sufficient relief a short sharp course of steroids is usually excellent at producing symptomatic relief. The regime often used for acute orchitis is recommended 40, 30, 20, 10, 5 mg of prednisolone daily over a 5-day course. There may be some shrinkage of the affected testis post-infection but even in the 20% or less where the infection is bilateral there is no evidence whatsoever of *reduced fertility*.

Other complications

All the salivary glands can be affected. Submandibular more common than submental. Pancreatitis is very rare and of the last 10 children admitted with mumps to the Regional Infectious Diseases Unit in Manchester suspected of having pancreatitis, nine were

constipated (probably secondary to the analgesia and mild dehydration) and the tenth had appendicitis and no evidence of
mumps at all.

Differential diagnosis

There are a number of other causes of parotid swelling, and
adenoviruses can cause an illness very similar to mumps. The older
the patient (over 40) the less likely the illness is to be mumps and
the geriatric patient especially is much more likely to have bacterial parotitis (usually caused by *Staphylococcus aureus* in a debilitated patient). Remember that mumps is a swelling of the face/
cheeks in which the patient loses the angle of the jaw, and the
major differential diagnosis of lymphadenopathy in that area most
often causes swelling of the neck, not face. Mumps is also an acute
febrile illness and the classic causes of chronic parotid swelling
such as tumour or sarcoidosis can also cause fever. Especially in
the older patient check the teeth and tonsils and ensure that the
swelling is in the parotid.

Mumps vaccination

This is not carried out in the United Kingdom because of the very
low mortality and morbidity of the illness. Mortality would normally be associated with encephalitis/meningitis (see Chapter 10).
Immunization uptake of less than 95% would only probably produce a larger susceptible adult population; the very group in which
most of the morbidity occurs.

GLANDULAR FEVER (infectious mononucleosis)

Glandular fever is caused by the Epstein–Barr virus, which is a
DNA virus of the herpes group. Most people in the United Kingdom will have been infected before they leave school or college,
and many even before they start school. The vast majority of
infections are subclinical. The United Kingdom general practitioner will be familiar with a typical clinical angiose glandular
fever: usually a teenager who has a markedly febrile illness, wide-

spread lymphadenopathy and very often a sore throat. Most cases recover spontaneously and all that is needed is symptomatic relief with antipyretic analgesia.

Epidemiology

The classical picture is commoner in the higher social classes (I and II), presumably because more crowded families in lower social classes have greater exposure before adolescence. The virus is not very tough and needs to be kept warm and wet but can be excreted from the throat for 18 months after an infection; hence, its 'kissing disease' tag. The incubation period is 1–2 months but can be much shorter if acquired from blood transfusion (a well-recorded but exceptionally rare event).

Diagnosis

The diagnosis is most easily confirmed by a simple blood count showing atypical monocytes and a positive monospot test. The monospot test works on the same principle as a Paul–Bunnell test – that is the fact that the heterophile antibodies do not react with guinea pig kidney cells. The monospot is a slide test instead of tube dilutions. The tests are very good and specific, and the main reason they are occasionally negative is that the antibodies do not appear until well into the second week of the illness.

Management

The commonest management problem is the severe sore throat which can be so swollen that obstruction of the airway is feared. This is the commonest reason for admitting a glandular fever patient to hospital. Initial treatment should be with aspirin gargles and more recently the oral rinse, Difflam (benzydamine hydrochloride) has had some success in reducing local symptoms. A short, sharp course of steroids is often very beneficial (40, 30, 20, 10 and 5 mg) over 5 days, but the general practitioner should consider hospital admission if steroids are going to be used as in severe cases tracheostomy or intubation has been necessary and close observation is therefore essential.

Antibiotics

Of cases with severe pharyngitis, due to glandular fever, admitted to hospital under EMD in the last 2 years, 25% also had an infection with beta-haemolytic streptococcus. The antibiotic of choice is erythromycin. There is no defence for a general practitioner who prescribes a semi-synthetic penicillin, e.g. ampicillin/amoxyl, for a teenager with a fever and a sore throat. If the patient has glandular fever he or she will almost certainly develop a florid rash usually 7–10 days after starting the antibiotic. In the United States of America the prescription of a semi-synthetic penicillin to patients with glandular fever is the subject of automatic financial compensation. The rash can be very severe and debilitary and is the second commonest reason why glandular fever patients are admitted to hospital. To use the reaction to ampicillin as a diagnostic test is like using a red hot poker to test for peripheral neuropathy.

Other complications

Splenomegaly

Approximately 50% of patients with classical glandular fever illness will have detectable splenomegaly. They must be warned to avoid trauma even of a minor nature, and contact sports are absolutely taboo until complete resolution. Ruptured spleen accounts for 15% of deaths from glandular fever (including people with malignancies).

Neurological

Post-infectious polyradiculopathy (Guillain–Barré syndrome) can follow glandular fever but a mononeuritis, e.g. transient VI or III cranial nerve palsies, occasionally occur. Encephalitis is also well-recognized but exceptionally rare.

Hepatitis

Biochemical hepatitis is very common but actual jaundice clinically detectable occurs in only approximately 20% of hospitalized patients. Hospitalized patients are of course the severe end of the spectrum. Occasionally the illness is indistinguishable clinically from hepatitis A (see Chapter 9).

Haematological complications

Occasionally haemolytic anaemia or thrombocytopenia complicate glandular fever. Both complications readily respond to steroid therapy.

Rash

An erythematous macular papular, urticarial or even purpuric rash can occur in its own right even without prior antibiotic treatment.

Tumours

Burkitt's lymphoma and oriental nasopharyngeal carcinoma are both associated with EBV but the association is unclear, and cause and effect are very much non-proven.

Immunosuppressed patients, and particularly patients with lymphoreticular malignancies, can have very severe, even fatal, infections with EBV.

Sore throat (angiose glandular fever)

It is clinically impossible to tell bad glandular fever from diphtheria so be particularly aware if the patient has recently been abroad. Thank goodness for the monospot test.

Chronic glandular fever

Glandular fever has a reputation for causing chronic tiredness and having a long convalescence. This occurs in a minority of patients (approximately 15%), and is probably due to a defect in 'T' cell lymphocytes. Eventual recovery after several months, as opposed to the few weeks in the 'normal' individual, is the rule.

The general practitioner is often confronted with a teenage patient suffering from glandular fever at examination times. Apart from general advice about plenty of rest and symptomatic relief of symptoms there is little a general practitioner can do. Steroid treatment is very occasionally helpful but should only be used, with specialist advice, for short periods.

A large dose of prednisolone (20–40 mg) has a brisk anti-inflammatory effect and usually makes the patient afebrile within 24 hours. It also reduces oedema in the pharynx to allow swallowing in relative comfort.

A large dose of steroids can have a beneficial effect on the patient's feeling of well-being. It can also have an unpleasant psychotic effect. Steroids, therefore, should not be given for the first time on the day of an examination.

For O-level examinations the large dose of steroid given the day before to the day after the examination may result in the patient being on 20 mg, or more, of prednisolone continuously for a month or longer. The risk of side-effects would therefore outweigh the advantages. O-levels could be taken again within a relatively short time without loss of general academic progress. A-levels and university finals are a different matter but are generally over a shorter period of time with fewer actual examination days. A more intermittent treatment is therefore possible with subsequent minimizing of side-effects.

Monospot negative glandular fever

Apart from the test being done too early there are two other infections which can be clinically very similar to EB virus infections:

(1) CMV (cytomegalovirus infection),

(2) toxoplasmosis.

Cytomegalovirus

This is another herpes virus and is widespread in the general population. Again most infections are asymptomatic, particularly when acquired very early in life. There is a peak of infection between 1 and 2 years old. The second peak of infection is between 15 and 30, when an illness similar to glandular fever can result. Splenomegaly, pharyngitis and general lymphadenopathy are much rarer, whereas frank hepatitis is more common. Cytomegalovirus infections can be very serious in two distinct situations; both will generally be out of the province of the general practitioner:

(1) Congenital infection - when acquired *in utero* severe damage can result and many die soon after birth. Unfortunately, unlike rubella, fetal infection can occur from reactivation as well as from primary infection (therefore the patient can have more than one child affected). However, half the congenitally infected children will show no signs at all, but most will have below-average mental development and many will have severe sensory-neural deafness.

(2) Cytomegalovirus is a patent cause of serious infection and death in transplant patients. It can be a reactivation of the patient's own virus or it may be present in the donor organ (particularly the kidneys). No effective, specific treatment is available as yet for cytomegalovirus infections although an acyclovar variant (pro-drug) has shown some promise.

TOXOPLASMOSIS

Toxoplasmosis is caused by the protozoan *Toxoplasma gondii*, which is widespread in nature. The reservoir of infection in the United Kingdom is the domestic cat.

As with Epstein–Barr virus (EBV) and cytomegalovirus (CMV) the majority of infections are subclinical and up to 50% of the adult population have serological evidence of infection without any known illness.

Epidemiology

The disease is acquired by eating cysts in raw or undercooked meat or food contaminated by cat faeces. At least one world-famous athlete no longer eats steak tartare after an episode of toxoplasmosis caused the loss of a prestigious championship.

Clinical features

Most cases seen by a general practitioner will present with lymphadenopathy. The presentation with malaise, fever and sore throat in addition is actually rare but must be remembered as a cause of monospot-negative glandular fever.

The majority of cases will settle spontaneously but persistent lymphadenopathy may lead to investigation and even biopsy.

Diagnosis

The diagnosis is confirmed in most cases by a rising titre or presence of IgM antibodies. A single titre of even 1/512 or 1/1024 is not diagnostic of recent infection.

Apart from glandular fever the other major differential is tuberculosis adenitis, particularly as the lymph nodes persist and are usually 'cold' and not tender. Occasionally a patient presents with retinitis or uveitis.

Similar to cytomegalovirus the protozoan can cause severe disease in two situations:

(1) congenital,

(2) immunocompromised.

Congenital toxoplasmosis

The organism crosses the placenta and an acute infection in pregnancy can lead to severe congenital toxoplasmosis. There is no risk of reactivation of latent infection and therefore congenital toxoplasmosis can only occur once in the progeny of one patient. The majority of infected infants will appear normal at birth but develop choroidoretinitis, mental retardation and epilepsy.

Immunocompromised toxoplasmosis

Toxoplasmosis can run a very virulent course in immunocompromised patients, most often by reactivations. The central nervous system is most often the site with encephalitis and cerebral abscesses but myocardial involvement (particularly in heart transplants) and pneumonitis can occur. *Toxoplasma* and the protozoan *Cryptospiridia* (see chapter on gastrointestinal infections) have increasingly been recognized as important opportunistic infections in patients suffering from AIDS (acquired immune deficiency syndrome).

Management

Most patients, even when the disease has been severe or chronic enough to result in investigation and therefore diagnosis, will *not* require any treatment.

Cotrimoxazole is probably the easiest treatment for a general practitioner to prescribe, and has been shown to have slight benefit when taken for 3 months. Pyrimethamine and sulphadiazine in combination for 1 month is the best oral treatment, but the role of folate supplements with this therapy needs resolution and often specialist advice is necessary. Spiramycin (also available parenterally) has been used with some success and is safer in pregnancy. Steroid treatment is important particularly when the eye is involved (with an inflammatory response).

Adequate cooking and the prevention of contamination of food by cat faeces is of course the best method of tackling the disease.

HERPES SIMPLEX

Herpes simplex infection is one of the commonest viral infections easily recognized in general practice, but most patients will not even present with the complaint of 'cold sores'. The common peri-oral lesions are seen frequently when patients are debilitated with other illnesses but occasionally the infection itself may be the reason for presentation.

Herpes simplex encephalitis is dealt with in the chapter on central nervous system infections and is fortunately rare, as it has a poor prognosis. Herpes simplex infections are generally divided into Herpes type I and Herpes type II. Herpes type II is most definitely a venereal infection (see Chapter 7) and the old adage 'type II below the waist type I above' still has some advantages, although in this promiscuous age it does not hold true completely.

Epidemiology

Most primary infections with the virus are subclinical, but it is spread readily by kissing, touch, droplet or even from drinking or eating utensils. Apart from the common cold sores there are several distinct clinical entities that are occasionally seen in general practice that deserve specific mention as their management is somewhat different.

Primary stomatitis

Primary stomatitis can occur at any age but is predominantly a pre-school child problem. The first sign is usually discrete oral ulceration in a child who has stopped eating, and over a few days the whole of the oral cavity can become ulcerated. The child is very miserable, febrile and has marked lymphadenopathy but above all has a very painful mouth which sometimes prevents the consumption of liquids as well as solids. Less severe episodes do, of course, occur.

After 4 or 5 days the lesions begin to crust and the patient slowly returns to normal. There is always significant weight loss but it is soon regained and the lymphadenopathy subsides in a few weeks.

Management

Adequate analgesia and the maintenance of fluid intake are the cornerstones of the management of stomatitis. The simple device of using a straw to drink with can be very effective, but the commonest reason for hospital admission is the lack of oral intake.

Specific anti-viral therapy using acyclovir is only justified in the minority of extreme cases or where an underlying problem (e.g. immunosuppression) is known. The lymphadenopathy should not be investigated unless it persists for many weeks. Primary herpetic stomatitis is *not* a presentation of patients with lymph node malignancies, although it does occur in patients known to have malignant disease.

Herpes simplex infection in the atopic eczema patient

Eczema herpeticum occurs in patients known to have severe eczema and is somewhat similar to the old-fashioned eczema vaccinatum. Herpes simplex infection spreads very easily over eczematous skin and is undoubtedly *made worse* by using local steroids.

The first time it occurs the infection can be very serious and life-threatening. The main danger to life is from secondary infection with *Staphylococcus aureus* or beta-haemolytic streptococcus group A causing septicaemia.

Hospital admission is usually necessary on the first occasion, but subsequent episodes are less serious. Any evidence of secondary infection should be treated with oral flucloxacillin or erythromycin in penicillin-sensitive patients.

Herpetic whitlow

Occasionally what appears to be a septic paronychia may fail to resolve with adequate antibiotic treatment (usually flucloxacillin). There may be easily indentifiable pus present but on culture it is sterile and sometimes recurrence occurs. It is an occupational hazard of intensive care nurses, and the patient does not very often have herpetic lesions elsewhere.

Treatment with idoxuridine (IDU) in dimethyl sulphoxide (DMSO) for 4 days, or 5% acyclovir cream until resolution, is sometimes necessary but often the lesions will clear spontaneously and the main reason for treatment is the prevention of other lesions, either in the patient themselves (particularly their eyes) or in their children or even patients in the care of the intensive care nurse. All lesions should be kept covered with secure fingerstall dressings until completely healed.

Herpes simplex infection of the eye

Herpetic keratoconjunctivitis is a rare but important infection of the eye. It usually presents with a unilateral painful red eye and is more common when 'cold sores' or where other herpes simplex infections are present.

Exclusion of an herpetic infection with its classical dendritic ulcer appearance is very important before using local steroids in any eye infection. Immunofluorescent 'dye' strips may allow easy visualization, but in certain circumstances slit-lamp examinations by ophthalmologists may be necessary.

Treatment

There are several local antiviral preparations; 5% idoxuridine (Kerocid) and 3% acyclovir (Zorvirax) are the commonest. The pain often resolves before the infection is cleared and most cases need treatment for at least a week, and many much longer.

Erytheme multiforme

Herpes simplex infections are the commonest cause of this unpleasant skin condition characterized by target lesions with circular erythematous lesions surrounding a paler area with an erythematous centre. Most of the skin is involved, including the palms of the hands and the soles of the feet, and blistering can be quite severe. A more severe form, affecting the mucous membranes of the mouth, eyes and genital tracts, is called Stevens–Johnston syndrome and can even be fatal.

Hospital admission for Stevens–Johnston syndrome is usually mandatory. Intravenous fluid is often necessary. Local treatment with bland, soothing creams and mouthwashes is helpful for symptomatic relief. Systemic steroids are often used and the most difficult complication of all is eye involvement which occasionally needs intraocular steroids.

The other major causes of erythema multiforme are mycoplasmal pneumonia and drug allergies. Sulphonamides are the most often incriminated, particularly since the advent of combination therapy like cotrimoxazol (sulphonamide plus trimethoprim).

A diligent search for *Mycoplasma* infection is worthwhile as specific therapy with erythromycin or tetracycline (in adults only) can shorten the illness. Remember that *Mycoplasma* is the commonest cause of atypical pneumonia, and chest physical signs and even symptoms can be completely absent (see Chapter 4).

The antimalarial prophylactic drug fansidar (see Chapter 13) has recently been partly withdrawn from recommendations because of a high incidence of Stevens–Johnston syndrome with some deaths, in the United States of America.

12

Skin Infections

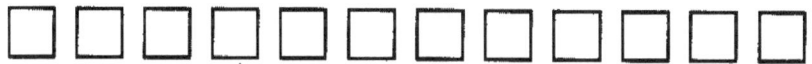

This chapter will include common infections of the eye and the external ear. Table 12.1 outlines a classification of infections commonly seen in general practice.

Table 12.1   Common skin infections in general practice

The ear	Otitis externa. Furunculosis
The eye	Conjunctivitis. Blepharitis. Dendritic ulcer. Stye (hordeolum). Chalazia. Lacrimal gland and duct infection (dacryocystitis)
The breast	Breast abscess
The hand	Paronychia. Pulp space infection
The genitalia	Balanoposthitis. Vulvitis. Bartholin abscess. Perianal abscess. Ischiorectal abscess
The feet	Fungus infections. Ingrowing toenail
The scalp	Pediculosis. Fungus infections. Bacterial infections
The skin	Impetigo, boils and carbuncles. Fungus infections. Infected sebaceous cysts. Infected eczema. Warts. Perianal eczema. Infestations

THE EAR – OTITIS EXTERNA AND FURUNCULOSIS

Otitis externa is a common problem in general practice. During a 12-month period in DB's practice there were 64 new episodes –

that is, 0.57% of all new episodes of illness – and the average general practitioner should meet one patient per fortnight.

The condition is not well understood and it is poorly managed in general practice. It has been classified as infective or reactive in that it may be primarily an infection, whether bacteriological, fungal or viral, or a manifestation of any other skin disorder such as eczema, seborrhoeic dermatitis or neurodermatitis which may have become secondarily infected. A furuncle is a staphylococcal infection of a hair follicle characterized by severe pain and localized swelling due to oedema. Otitis externa is more diffuse but can be equally painful. Both present similarly and on examination the meatal skin is red, swollen and tender. In furunculosis or otitis externa, pain may be produced by moving the jaw or pressing the tragus or pulling the pinna upwards.

Management

In the acute stage the most crucial and most neglected part of treatment is the meticulous cleansing of the meatus. Hicks (1983) demonstrated the importance of this in a small series of general practice cases, not only in terms of rapid resolution, but also in the differential diagnosis of serious attic perforations. Cotton wool, Jobson Horne probe, adequate vision and 12 mm ribbon gauze impregnated with Vioform-hydrocortisone cream are ideal. In the more chronic phase, framycetin and hydrocortisone acetate ear drops (Framycort) are helpful. In the presence of a drum perforation, framycetin, gentamicin and neomycin are best avoided because of the possibility of inducing permanent deafness. Alternative preparations include clioquinol and flumethasone pivalate 0.02% (Locorten; Vioform) and aluminium acetate ear drops. Ear drops are supplied in 10 ml quantities and applied three or four times daily.

Systemic antibiotics

Systemic antibiotics are advisable when there is marked oedema or adenitis. *Pseudomonas pyocyaneus*, *Bacillus proteus* and *Staphylococcus aureus* are common infecting organisms. Flucloxacillin (Floxapen) is a useful preparation in a dose of 250 g q.d.s.

Failure to respond

Common reasons for failure to respond include the presence of an underlying suppurative otitis media, fungal infection, skin sensitization to the topical application being used and persistence of a basic neurodermatitis associated with an intractable psychosomatic disturbance. *Aspergillus niger* and *Candida albicans* fungus infections may be treated by nystatin powder or ointment or amphotericin B (Fungilin) drops. Treatment should be continued for at least a week after apparent resolution. Herpes zoster and herpes simplex may occasionally involve the external ear.

THE EYE – CONJUNCTIVITIS AND DENDRITIC ULCERS

Acute infective conjunctivitis and small corneal ulcers respond well to treatment. Drops are probably better for conjunctivitis and ointment is probably better for ulcers. Chloramphenicol or neomycin eye ointment or drops both have a wide spectrum of activity and should be used first at least 4-hourly during the day. Aetiology is varied – viruses, *H. influenzae*, *S. aureus* and *Streptococcus viridans* commonly being isolated. In recent years *chlamydia trachomatis* has been detected more frequently and accounts for many infections resistant to chloramphenicol. Ophthalmia neonatonum due to gonococcus is extremely rare in general practice.

Blepharitis

This chronic and recurrent infection of the eyelids is often associated with scalp seborrhoea and may also have an allergic component. Steroid antibiotic ointment – framycetin sulphate, hydrocortisone acetate (Framygen) – applied four times daily is helpful. Staphylococcal blepharitis is ulcerated and responds to an antibiotic such as chloramphenicol eye ointment.

Styes (hordeolum) and chalazia

A chalazion or meibomian cyst is a granuloma occurring in a meibomian gland. If it should become painful, abscess formation has occurred. Systemic penicillin may be needed but incision and curettage will ultimately be required. Styes can be differentiated from chalazia because they point at the lid margin; a stye is an abscess in one of the glands related to a lash follicle. Systemic penicillin may be needed for crops but chloramphenicol eye ointment will often suffice.

Dacryocystitis

Infection of the nasolachrymal duct presents as an acute swelling on the inner corner of the eye and is often associated with systemic upset. Systemic penicillin should be given but incision and drainage may be required.

THE BREAST

Breast abscesses

Breast abscesses are seen less frequently than they used to be. This is probably the result of better antenatal care in that prevention of engorgement, nipple toilet and prompt therapy have prevented the development of the enormous abscesses which used to require drainage in the Casualty Department.

When they do occur, abscesses develop most commonly in the lactating breast, the responsible organism (usually *S. aureus*) gaining entry through a cracked nipple. The first response is a cellulitis which will respond to antibiotics. Flucloxacillin orally or parenteral penicillin should be first choice therapy, but erythromycin is a useful alternative in the presence of penicillin allergy.

If there is no response after 48 hours or if the infection is established when first seen, immediate admission is necessary so that the abscess might be drained. If the abscess is fluctuant, breast damage has already occurred.

Conflicting advice is often found about breast feeding. If the infection is treated with antibiotics in general practice, lactation can, if desired, be continued and milk expressed manually.

THE HAND

Paronychia

Paronychia is common in general practice and may be acute or chronic.

Acute paronychia

This is characterized by the sudden development of an acute painful swelling around a nailfold, often involving the forefinger. The responsible organism is usually *S. aureus* and entry is gained via a cuticle damaged by frequent wetting or inappropriate manicure. Early infections may be aborted by flucloxacillin or erythromycin but established infections may well require surgery. An occupational herpetic whitlow is not uncommon in nurses.

Chronic paronychia

In chronic paronychia the organisms involved vary, and include herpes virus, but they do evoke a much less pronounced tissue response and there is much more emphasis on provoking factors such as constant wetting which allows *C. albicans* and other bacteria to gain entry to the potential space between the nailfold and the underlying nail. Housewives and thumb-sucking children are common victims to an intermittent chronic painful swelling around the nail which discharges intermittently. The nail may well become deformed as a result of damage to the proximal nailfold.

It is important that the fingers be kept dry. Oral erythromycin and nystatin ointment applied three or four times daily are the most effective treatment.

Pulp space infections

These are most uncommon in general practice and require expert surgical treatment when they occur.

THE GENITALIA

Balanoposthitis

Balanoposthitis is the term given to infection of the foreskin and glans penis. The causative organisms in adults have been variously reported as *Candida* spp., group B streptococci, herpes simplex virus and *trichomonas vaginalis*, but over the past couple of decades the importance of anaerobic infection has become increasingly recognized.

In general practice the infection is common in young boys because of an associated ammoniacal dermatitis, and the diagnosis is easily made from the red excoriated appearance of the glans and foreskin, often with a purulent discharge. Poor hygiene can be an associated factor.

Many cases respond readily to local hygiene and bland creams such as Unguentum Merck or E45 cream but, when local hygiene is not sufficient, oral antibiotics, nystatin cream, antiseptic creams, e.g. chlorhexidine (Hibitane), or metronidazole may be needed depending on causative factors and age. Do remember in adults that resistant cases may be associated with an underlying cause such as diabetes.

Bartholin abscess

A Bartholin abscess is relatively uncommon in general practice and results from infection of a Bartholin cyst which has developed as a result of a congenital or acquired abnormality of the Bartholin duct.

Antibiotics rarely work and the diagnosis should be considered a gynaecological emergency and the patient admitted for a marsupialization procedure.

Perianal abscess

An abscess beneath the perianal skin usually results from a sinus entering from a fissure *in ano*, a pilonidal sinus or an abscess of Cowper's gland. Antibiotic therapy with flucloxacillin and/or simple surgical incision is usually adequate therapy although on occasion, if the condition recurs frequently, referral may be necessary. Do not forget that ischaemic bowel disease may occasionally present this way.

Ischiorectal abscess

In the case of an ischiorectal abscess - rare in general practice - constitutional symptoms are severe and hospital admission is necessary.

THE FEET

Deep infections of the foot are rare in general practice (compare with deep infections of the hand) and require skilled treatment in hospital.

Superficial infections are common, however.

Ingrowing toe nail

The nailfold of the great toe may become traumatized by a sharp nail due to poor nail trimming. This can become infected and a granulomatous overgrowth then gives the impression of an ingrowing toenail. Chiropody surgery is often necessary but early lesions may well respond to local hygiene. Alcoholic iodine solution can be painted on with cotton wool swabs and is helpful in some cases.

Tinea pedis

The feet are a common site for infection with fungal organisms, such as *Trichophyton rubrum*. It has been suggested that half the population have tinea pedis at some time in their life. Characteristically there is an erythamatosquamous rash and possibly small vesicles, especially between the toes and over the instep. Peeling maceration and fissuring may follow. Severe itching is a predominant symptom but it should be remembered that other lesions will also be termed 'athlete's foot' by the patient, such as eczema

- whether enogenous or due to shoe dyes, psoriasis, bacterial infections and candidal infections.

The tinea infections involve the feet because of the moist warm environment that encourages spread. Swimming baths, changing room showers and squash clubs and badminton clubs are common sources of infection.

Diagnois can often be made clinically but is best made from the microscopic examination of skin scrapings placed on a drop of potassium hydroxide on a slide, because treatment may need to be persistent and confident therapy requires firm diagnosis.

The first point in management is to keep the feet dry. Shoes should be porous, sock changes should be frequent and an anti-fungal foot powder such as Mycil powder may be helpful.

Single patches are best treated by compound benzoic acid oint-ment (Whitfield's ointment), tolnaftate (Tinaderm), clotrimazole (Canestan) or miconazole nitrate (Daktarin). Oral griseofulvin is only used if there is associated toenail infection.

SKIN INFECTIONS

Normal skin flora

At the moment of birth the skin of the newborn baby is colonized by non-pathogenic staphylococci and diptheroids, which are the two predominant organisms on the skin of the adult. *S. aureus* and other pathogens may also be cultured from the skin of normal people but healthy intact skin is very resistant to infection and succumbs only in the presence of a virulent strain, mechanical disruption to the skin (abrasions, cracks, inflammation), the use of corticosteroids, lower body resistance (diabetes) or immune deficiency. Bacteria, fungi, yeasts and viruses may be involved.

Impetigo

The patients are usually children and the causative organism is *S. aureus*. The lesion is characterized by superficial thin-walled blis-ters which rupture easily leaving a yellowish exudate and crusts, especially on the face, but the scalp, buttocks and hands may also be involved. It should be remembered that impetigo may be a secondary as well as a primary infection and may follow eczema or scabies and render the primary condition resistant to treatment.

Antibiotics applied topically are very effective because of the superficial nature of the lesion. Gentamicin (Cidomycin; Genticin), neomycin or fusidate (Fucidin) ointment applied three or four times daily are useful. If impetigo is widespread, systemic antibiotics are needed, preferably flucloxacillin (Floxapen) or erythromycin. Very rarely the streptococcus may be involved and even more rarely nephritis has been reported as a consequence.

Boils, folliculitis, carbuncles

A boil or furuncle is caused by the invasion of a hair follicle with *S. aureus*. Folliculitis is the name given to the multiple small pustular lesions centred on hair follicles on the beard or the thighs, and a carbuncle is a collection of boils which have localized to form a deeper, more extensive lesion which is indurated and pustular.

Systemic flucloxacillin or erythromycin should be given if there is surrounding cellulitis, but if a boil is well localized simple heat may suffice; incision and drainage are usually required at some stage, particularly if the boil is throbbing and painful.

Recurrent boils are troublesome and, despite the stories in the textbooks, do not seem to be associated in clinical practice with covert diabetes. There is usually a source of infection such as the nares, otitis externa or perianal eczema and general body defences may be lowered for many reasons ranging from simple stress or depression to overt infection. Crops of boils in the axillae require antibiotic therapy and occasionally referral for excision of the apocrine gland bearing area.

Streptococcal infections

Streptococcal infection of the skin is relatively rare in general practice but erysipelas due to the β-haemolytic streptococcus is seen from time to time. It is often preceded by an upper respiratory infection and commonly involves the legs as a result of degenerative skin changes in older people. Lymphatic spread is characteristic. There may be general symptoms of headache, malaise, feverishness and vomiting. The spreading edge of the rash is clearly defined.

The treatment of choice is penicillin. Severe attacks require parenteral benzylpenicillin 0.5 megaunits i.m. 6-hourly for 5 days, but in general practice the condition is usually treated early with penicillin V 250–500 mg 6-hourly. Desquamation and pigmentation may persist for some time and elastic stockings may be helpful until lymphatic drainage is resolved.

Fungal infections

The classification of fungal infections is complicated and insecure. Three major genera of ringworm fungi can infect man, namely *Microsporum*, *Epidermophyton* and *Trichophyton*. These have been divided yet again by cultural characteristics into numerous species, some of which produce specific forms of disease. Infection with fungal organisms may be superficial (skin, nails and hair) or deep, and there is marked geographical variation. For example, *Trichophyton rubrum* infection of the feet and nails now predominates in the UK, while scalp ringworm is rare.

Epidemiology

About half the known species of dermatophytes are transferred from man to man and do not infect animals. The rest originate from animals or the soil. Cutaneous candidiasis and tinea versicolor form separate groups of superficial infections. Susceptibility is influenced by a number of factors including heredity, an animal reservoir, congested living conditions, swimming pools and immigration which may bring new species.

Tinea capitis

Scalp ringworm is rare in Britain at the present time. *Microsporum audouini* is a human pathogen whereas *Microsporum canis* is an animal species passed on from cats and dogs. It is largely a problem involving pre-pubertal children in whom any bald patches accompanied by scaling and broken-off hairs must be assumed to be tinea capitis until proved otherwise. Oral griseofulvin and local antifungal agents are advisable.

Tinea barbae

This is rare and is easily confused with folliculitis barbae. Steroid cream should not be prescribed just because a presumed bacterial infection does not clear up.

Tinea corporis

This is common and presents in various ways including reddish papules, annular and circinate lesions with scaling and an advancing raised peripheral border with central healing.

Tinea cruris

This is particularly common in males and the lower abdomen and inner thighs may be involved as well as the groins. Tinea pedis commonly coexists. Predisposing factors include sweating, obesity, tight athletic supports and a hot climate. *Trichophyton* spp. and *Epidermophyton* spp. may both be responsible and both respond to systemic griseofulvin, although local treatment may be adequate.

Nail ringworm (tinea unguium)

Infection with *T. rubrum* is probably the commonest nail disorder. The toenails are almost always affected and a brownish-yellow discoloration may be the only obvious sign. Softening, fragility and irregular thickening follow. Therapy is not always needed, but women and all with fingernail involvement may prefer treatment. Oral griseofulvin 500 mg daily until all the infected tissue has been shed may need 9 months or less in fingernail disease or 12–18 months in toenail disease. Relapse or failure is common. Modern topical agents may be helpful.

Tinea versicolor

Tinea versicolor is a superficial skin infection caused by a yeast-like fungus characterized by light-brown or white, slightly scaly lesions on the chest, trunk and neck; lesions are particularly obvious after exposure to the sun as the areas do not tan. Even after cure, pigmentation may take a little while to return. The causative organism is *Malassezia furfur*.

The condition responds well to many topical antifungal agents. Sodium thiosulphate, compound benzoic acid ointment, clotrimazole (Canestan) and miconazole nitrate (Daktarin) cream and selenium sulphide suspension (Selsun) shampoo applications all produce rapid improvement. The recurrence rate is reduced by protracted courses of treatment.

Candida infections

Candida species (usually *C. albicans*) may exist as harmless saprophytes in the vagina, the gastrointestinal and respiratory tracts and the exposed surface of normal skin. It is therefore likely that predisposing factors contribute to the development of acute and chronic infection. These include a moist warm environment, the pathogenicity of the species, diabetes mellitus, underlying disease of the lymphoreticular system, antibacterial chemotherapy, the use of corticosteroids (systemic and topical) and immunosuppressive agents. Candidiasis is more common in infants, the elderly and in women. Superficial candidiasis affects the skin (paronychia, intertriginous, perianal and generalized cutaneous forms) and mucous membranes (oral angular stomatitis, vulvovaginitis and balanitis).

Treatment of fungal diseases

Yeast infections caused by *C. albicans* respond to topical applications of nystatin (Nystan), amphotericin B (Fungilin) or clotrimazole (Canestan). Gentian violet, though effective, is usually cosmetically unacceptable. Twice-daily applications should be continued for at least 2–3 weeks for skin candidiasis and 4–6 weeks for chronic candidal paronychia.

Dermatophyte infections are best treated with griseofulvin (Grisovin; Fulcin) 500 mg daily taken with a fatty meal. Duration of therapy depends on clearance times. Tinea corporis requires 3-4 weeks, tinea capitis 3-5 weeks, palms 6 weeks, soles 6-8 weeks, fingernails 3-9 months, toenails 1-2 years and toe webs 4-6 weeks.

Topical application does have a place in the treatment of superficial fungal infection. Single patches of ringworm and toe web infections are suitable for treatment with compound benzoic acid ointment (Whitfield's ointment), tolnaftate (Tinaderm), clotrimazole (Canestan) or miconazole nitrate (Daktarin). This approach may well be good enough for tinea cruris, although the relapse rate is lower if systemic treatment is used as well. Griseofulvin is very safe but diarrhoea is an occasional complication. Tinea versicolor does not respond to griseofulvin. Chronic candidal paronychia, intertriginous, perianal and napkin candidiasis respond well to topical nystatin cream, Candida vulvovaginitis has been described elsewhere (p. 89).

Perianal eczema (pruritus ani)

This is such a common problem in general practice that it deserves a separate description. Pruritus ani is part dermatological, part psychological, occasionally proctological and commonly infective. The first essential is skin trauma which is often due to vigorous attempts to cleanse the perianal skin with paper or attempts to scratch an area rendered pruritic as a result of psychological stress. Predisposing tendencies include vaginal discharge, urinary leakage, excessive sweating, mucous anal discharge with third degree piles, perianal sepsis, fistula *in ano*, chronic diarrhoea and tight underclothes, especially of the nylon variety. Diabetes, worms (see p. 133) and a susceptibility to fungal infection may also be relevant.

When skin defences have been broken, further scratching will compound the problem and infection with saprophytic bacteria and fungi is inevitable. The byproducts of micro-organisms may then induce an allergic response which further complicates management.

Particular management problems are produced by perianal polypharmacy often containing steroids, local anaesthetics, antibiotics and a greasy base, which are frequent causes in themselves of skin sensitivity. Topical steroids make fungal overgrowth more likely. If they are used at all, treatment of this sort should be limited to 1 week.

The essential component of treatment is to keep the perianal skin scrupulously clean and protected from physical trauma. Ideally one should wash with a jet of water, a moist cloth or cotton wool. Baby wipes are ideal for this purpose and remove residual faecal material which provokes the continuing problem.

Non-porous clothing in order to maintain a dry perianal skin is next, and in this context astringent lotions may be helpful, such as 0.5% aqueous solution of silver nitrate. Antifungal creams may be helpful if fungal infection is suspected.

Warts

Common warts are caused by skin infection with the wart virus. There are a number of morphological types. Plantar warts involve the soles of the feet, filiform warts are often seen on the head and neck. Flat (plane) warts are discrete, often multiple, lesions on the face or backs of the hands. Penile or vulval warts may be papillomatous or acuminate. Periungual warts are usually multiple and are common in nail biters.

Destructive measures are necessary for treatment. Topical applications of strong acids, formaldehyde solution, podophyllin and salicylic acid in solution or in the form of plasters are safe and usually successful as long as instructions are followed. Liquid nitrogen or carbon dioxide snow are more painful and require skilled supervision. Plantar warts respond best when chiropody surgery is involved at the same time.

SKIN INFESTATION

Ectoparasites are common. Indeed, up to 5% of patients referred to dermatology clinics are said to have this problem. Classification includes zoonoses from domestic animals, human scabies, pediculosis and finally other acarine dermatoses caused by acari in stored foods, house and other dusts. Table 12.2 presents the causes of infestations in man.

Table 12.2 Infestations in man

Causes of infestation*	Sources
Order Hymenoptera (bees, wasps, hornets and ants)	
Order Diptera (mosquitoes, gnats, midges and horse flies)	
Order Syphonaptera (fleas)	Dogs, cats, hedgehogs, rabbits, man
Order Hemiptera (bedbugs)	Man
Order Anoplura (lice)	Man
Sarcoptes scabiei (human)	Human
Sarcoptes scabiei (animal)	Dogs, horses, camels etc
Cheyletiella spp	Dogs, cats, rabbits
Dermanyssus gallinae	Fowl
Dermanyssus hirundinis	Cage birds, swallows
Ophyoniassus natricis	Snakes
Acarus siro	Foods
Tyrophagus spp	Foods
Glycyphagus spp	Dusts
Dermatophagoides pteronyssimus	Dusts
Dermatophagoides farinae	Dusts
Trombicula autumnalis	Vegetation
Pyemotes spp	Vegetation, grain, wood

* The most important groups are underlined. (From Hewitt, 1975)

The reaction

Flea punctures produce groups of erythematous macules, often with a visible central puncture. Weals and excoriations are common and the lesion irritates. Papules are very common and papular urticaria is a common sign of flea infestation in children. Lengthy exposure in all age groups can lead to secondary pigmentation eczema and infection.

Animal scabies

Dogs, pigs, horses, sheep, goats and other mammals can all be infested with host-specific *Sarcoptes scabiei*. About 1% of all dogs are infested and scabies is seen on the face, ear flaps, limbs and groin. The parasite can produce a contact dermatois in man. A papular rash develops in a few hours at the site of contact, lower legs, thighs, lower abdomen and the flexoral aspects of the forearm. The lesions itch when the patient is hot. There are no burrows and papular lesions may affect the face. There may be generalized erythema eczematization and pigmentation.

Management

Benzyl benzoate is only partly effective. Crotamiton 10% cream (Eurax) may relieve the irritation. Veterinary advice is needed and the Environmental Health Officer should be informed.

Human scabies

Up-to-date figures for infestation with human scabies do not exist. Presentation used to be in the form of epidemics and the condition is pandemic in India and South America. Infection occurs through close body contact and is frequently venereally acquired. Only rarely is scabies transmitted through bedclothes but it can be transmitted from patients to nursing staff, particularly in overcrowded geriatric units. Norwegian crusted scabies is a rare infestation with *S. scabiei* var. *hominis* which tends to occur in mentally defective and debilitated patients. Thick crusted lesions like psoriasis are found on the limbs and trunk. Medicated soaps (Tetmosol) can be useful in institutions.

The reaction

The lesions are characterized by burrows. Ninety per cent of patients have burrows in interdigital spaces, palms, flexoral surfaces of wrists and the ulnar border of the hands. Other areas include the forearms, navel, external genitals and buttocks.

Management

It is important that applications be used on the entire skin surface of the infested patient from the chin to the soles of the feet, otherwise immature mites could be missed. All members of the household and all close contacts must be treated at the same time. Benzyl benzoate application B.P. is the treatment of choice and is best applied with a 1-inch or 2-inch paintbrush. Less irritant preparations include 1% gamma benzine hexachloride cream (Lorexane) or lotion (Quellada); monosulphiram (Tetmosol) 25% solution diluted with about three parts water before use, and crotamiton (Eurax) lotion or ointment. Table 12.3 shows a routine for treatment. Residual irritation may last a few weeks.

Table 12.3   Treatment of scabies

Day 1
(1)   Hot bath using soap and rub skin gently with a flannel, particularly at the sites of the burrows
(2)   Dry with a towel
(3)   Apply the preparation to the whole of the body from the chin to the soles of the feet. Let it dry on the skin
(4)   Go to bed; the preparation on the skin will kill any mites in the bedding

Day 2
Repeat the application without the hot bath.

Day 3
Wash off the preparation by bathing. Any residual irritation can be eased by crotamiton cream

All intimate contacts of the patient should undergo the same treatment

This treatment should be carried out even if there is eczematization and secondary infection. Often no further treatment is required. If itching continues after a month it usually indicates reinfection from an untreated contact, inadequate treatment of the previous attack, or incorrect diagnosis. In heavily infested closed communities the use of Tetmosol soap may help to prevent spread to others

---

(From Hewitt, 1975)

Pediculosis

Lice can affect man on the head (*Pediculus humanus capitis*), on the body (*Pediculus humanus corporis*) and in the pubic area (*Phthirus pubis*). They are wingless host specific insects which are usually recognized by their eggs (nits) and still occur in the heads of up to 10% of all schoolchildren in urban areas.

Body lice are rare except in tramps and in homes with extremely poor standards of hygiene. Pubic lice are a different genus and may also be found on the eyebrows or underarm hair. They are usually spread by direct contact but can be acquired from clothing or lavatory seats.

The reaction

The cardinal symptom is irritation and all children who scratch their heads require careful examination for lice.

Management

Management involves careful hygiene and treatment of all contacts. Regular bathing for *P. corporis* and *P. pubis* infestation with changes of underwear and application of gamma benzine hexachloride B.P.C. 1% cream (Lorexane) to the affected areas twice weekly. There is a shampoo (Lorexane No. 3) which is particularly useful for *P. capitis* infestation. Alternatives for capitis infestation include Lorexane cream which can be massaged into the scalp for 24 hours and Quellada application PC which contains gamma benzine hexachloride 1% in a shampoo base. After repeat applications in 7 days the hair can be shampooed normally.

REFERENCES AND FURTHER READING

Hewitt, M. (1975). Infestations of the skin. *Medicine (London)*, **32,** 1849
Hicks, S. C. (1983). Otitis externa: are we giving adequate care? *J. R. Coll. Gen. Practit.*, **33,** 581
Sarkany Imrich (1975). Infections of the skin. *Medicine (London)*, **32,** 1828

13

Imported Infections

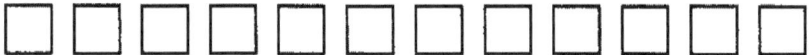

In 1984 over 5 million inhabitants of the UK had holidays in Spain alone. Very many others visited other Mediterranean countries. Foreign holidays in search of some summer sunshine have become commonplace. 'Have you been abroad recently?' is a very important question but is all too often forgotten. The patient most at risk is not the holidaymaker with the telltale suntan but the businessman or engineer who has made the working trip to exotic parts.

Unexplained fevers and/or diarrhoea are the commonest problems brought to an infectious diseases unit. But Reid and colleagues[1] have shown that *respiratory* symptoms are the commonest on return to Glasgow.

Jaundice, general malaise, neurological symptoms and rashes are the other main groups of presenting symptoms.

FEVER

Most of the common causes of febrile illnesses in Britain are just as common in other countries. The child with fever and cough from the international airport is just as likely to have measles or influenza as malaria or typhoid.

Malaria

Human malaria can be divided into two main groups. *Plasmodium falciparum* malaria is life-threatening and still kills regularly in the United Kingdom. In 1983 12 people died and for the fifth year in succession death from undiagnosed malaria was the subject of a substantial settlement by the Medical Defence Societies. *Plasmodium vivax*, *P. ovale* and *P. malariae* are more benign and come into the category of a mild febrile illness and vague ill health.

Size of problem

More cases of malaria than of bacterial meningitis were notified in the UK in 1983 (approximately 1400 v. 1200). This actually represents a drop in the total number of cases of malaria from a high of 2000 in 1980.

The disappointing aspect is that the total number of falciparum cases, 441, was again an increase.

Diagnosis

Any patient returning from a tropical, or subtropical, area who becomes ill after return deserves the benefit of a malaria screen blood film. Malaria presents, usually, with fever and chills, sometimes even classical rigors with uncontrollable shaking. It can also present like hepatitis. Of patients with falciparum malaria, 40% give a significant history of diarrhoea. Very many have a cough, and an important few present with confusion alone. At least two people have died in recent years having been admitted to a psychiatric ward where the diagnosis of cerebral malaria was only made at postmortem. Physical signs are usually absent. Splenomegaly is uncommon and a tinge of jaundice is often very difficult to detect. The classic textbook periodicity of the fever is exceptionally rare.

In the last 200 cases seen over the past 10 years by EMD the 'fever every third day' pattern has only been seen once.

Treatment

Treatment depends upon the type of malaria and the treatment of the potentially life-threatening falciparum depends upon the areas visited. Chloroquine resistant falciparum is spreading rapidly and any cases from South America, south-east Asia, and now including Bangladesh and India and most of East and Central Africa, should be treated as chloroquine resistant.

Figure 13.1 shows areas of chloroquine resistance.

Anybody who is ill having returned from these places needs an urgent malaria film and probably hospital admission for treatment with combinations of quinine and Fansidar (pyrimethamine and sulphadoxone). Falciparum from West Africa can still be treated with chloroquine – four tablets (155 mg base) stat., two tablets 6 hours later and two tablets a day for 2 days.

Many patients who are visitors from West Africa would expect to be given the pills and leave the surgery to go home. This should only be done in exceptional circumstances. The commonest problem presented to EMD is a telephone call:

'I saw Mr X this morning, he's just back from Y and I thought he had malaria. I sent a blood sample to the lab and they say he's got malaria.'
EMD: 'What type?'
'I don't know.'
EMD: 'Where is the patient?'
'Gone home. No, he doesn't have a phone. Yes, I know it's 5 p.m. on Friday of a Bank Holiday weekend.'

If you are going to do an outpatient blood film the patient must be well and specific arrangements should be made to review, either in the evening surgery (if seen in the morning) or the following morning if seen in the evening.

The problems of outpatient films is that EDTA bottled samples if left more than a few hours will make malaria parasites more difficult to see. Machine-made films with bulk staining are not very suitable for the examination of parasites and many laboratories will do special stains and look hard if communicated with directly.

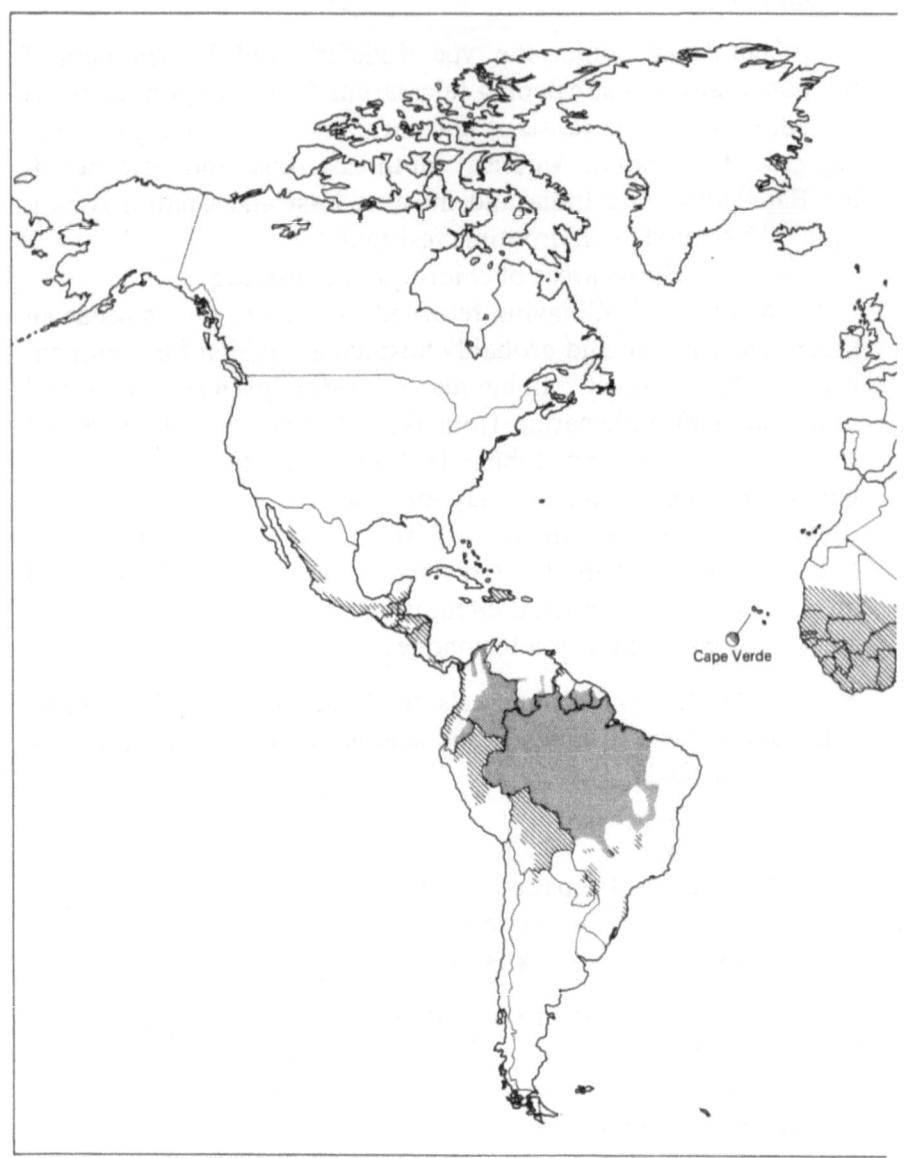

Figure 13.1 Epidemiological assessment of status of malaria, 1982

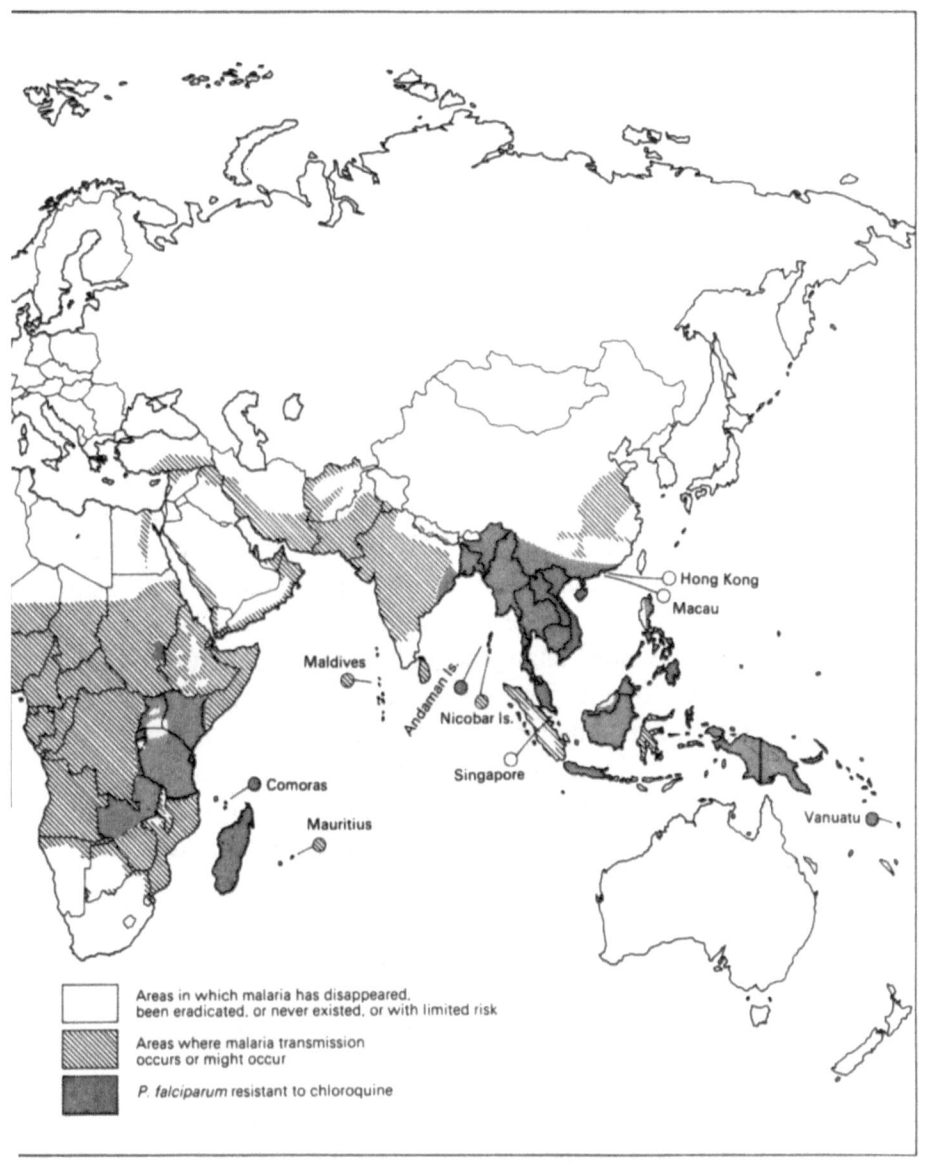

Areas in which malaria has disappeared, been eradicated, or never existed, or with limited risk

Areas where malaria transmission occurs or might occur

P. falciparum resistant to chloroquine

A short course of chloroquine for *P. vivax* and *P. ovale* should be followed by 14 days primaquine (15 mg per day for adults), to eradicate the ex-erythrocytic stages and prevent relapses. It is questionable whether primaquine is necessary for *P. malariae*.

Primaquine can cause severe haemolytic anaemia in G6PD deficient people. G6PD is sex-linked and occurs almost exclusively in males. It is commonest in the black races but all races have a variation and the type found in the semitic peoples can be severe.

Prophylaxis

Prophylaxis is difficult in the 1980s because of the changing resistant patterns. In areas of chloroquine resistant falciparum malaria, weekly Fansidar (pyrimethamine and sulphadoxone) or weekly Maloprim (pyrimethamine and dapsone) is probably best *added* to daily Paludrine (proguanil HCl) (200 mg or two tablets per day). Weekly chloroquine is still very effective (300 mg of base) in West Africa, Pakistan, western India and Sri Lanka.

This pattern may well change over the 1980s and up-to-date advice should be sought. The spread of chloroquine resistance throughout the Indian subcontinent is expected.

Prophylaxis for children is very difficult as only chloroquine is currently available in syrup form and even that is very bitter to taste. In general children over 12 should be given the adult dose (Table 13.1).

Table 13.1 Recommended doses of antimalarial drugs for prophylaxis in childhood[2]

Age	Chloroquine; proguanil	Fansidar; Maloprim
0–5 weeks	⅛ adult dose	Not recommended
6 weeks–5 months	¼ adult dose	⅛ adult dose
6 months–1 year	¼ adult dose	¼ adult dose
1–5 years (5–20 kg)	½ adult dose	½ adult dose
6–12 years (20–40 kg)	¾ adult dose	¾ adult dose
Over 12 years (40 kg)	Adult dose	Adult dose

Table 13.1 should, however, be used as only a rough guide. Only Fansidar tablets are easily split into quarters.

Daraprine (pyrimethamine alone) is no longer effective anywhere, but can still be bought over the counter at chemist's shops.

Pregnancy

Malaria is specially hazardous in pregnancy[3]. Paludrine is generally considered safe; chloroquine in normal prophylactic doses is also safe – it has caused several problems in the past when used for treating collagen diseases, but much higher doses were used.

Maloprim and Fansidar are considered unsafe in the first trimester and last 2 weeks.

Typhoid enteric fevers

Typhoid fever is the next most important imported infection in the United Kingdom and presents very much like malaria, i.e. as a pyrexia of unknown origin (*PUO*) with headache and rigors. There are between 150 and 200 cases per year (10% of the number of malaria cases). A number of these cases are of paratyphoid A and B (approximately 30%) and it must be remembered that approximately 15% are *not* imported at all.

Of the remaining 80–120 cases (depending on which year) the majority come from India, Pakistan and Africa. Approximately 15% only come from the Mediterranean holiday areas (the same number as the indigenous).

Diagnosis

Typhoid fever should be suspected in anyone who is ill with fever and headache within 14 days of return. They often have abdominal pain and are constipated and many are initially sent to hospital as possible cases of appendicitis. Provided that the patient doesn't continue to the diarrhoeal phase on a general surgery ward this does very little harm but usually delays treatment for 3–4 days. The mortality of typhoid fever, however, is increased approximately 50% if laparotomy is undertaken, but this probably reflects the fact that the more severe cases undergo laparotomy. The mortality is now much less than the pre-antibiotic figures of 15-20% and of the last 200 cases treated in the Regional Infectious Diseases Unit in Manchester only one has died (from severe haemorrhage).

Clinical picture

The patient often looks apathetic and ill with a high fever and a relative bradycardia. A non-productive cough is present in many and most are constipated in the early stages.

Unfortunately paediatric typhoid often presents like gastro-enteritis and children often have diarrhoea and vomiting (plus fever).

The famous 'rose spots' are not very useful to general practitioners. They are pale-pink, blanch on pressure and are usually clustered round the lower thorax and upper abdomen. They are probably present in more than the reported 10% but are usually difficult to see on suntanned or naturally black or brown skins.

Treatment

Hospital admission is usually mandatory to confirm the diagnosis. The best confirmation is by *positive* blood culture but in the very early stages the faeces are often positive as well and this should *not* be taken to mean the patient is a carrier.

Treatment is usually with chloramphenicol or co-trimoxazole. Ampicillin and mensillinan have not found the favour in the UK that they have elsewhere. A significant relapse rate within 3-4 weeks is not uncommon.

Carriers

General practitioners usually have difficulties after the diagnosis is suspected and the patients not admitted to hospital are usually carriers. Carriers should not be food handlers on discharge. Carriers should not be confused with convalescent excretors. Only a small proportion of convalescent excretors will become carriers.

The carrier state is often associated with gallbladder disease but cholecystectomy is very much rarer in Britain than in the USA. Cholecystectomy still carries a significant mortality and morbidity on both sides of the Atlantic and should not be carried out lightly.

Patient returning from abroad with diarrhoea

The management of a patient recently returned from abroad with diarrhoea varies very little from that which applies to a patient who has not left the United Kingdom (Chapter 8).

Most will have self-limiting causes and initial investigation will probably be limited to food handlers (remember to include air hostesses) and if the diarrhoea fails to settle quickly (a day or two) stool culture should be accompanied by microscopy for amoebae and *giardia lamblia*.

Any illness which is even a little more than an ordinary 'tummy bug' should be investigated if the patient has come from the tropics and the threshold for hospital admission should probably be a little lower than normal even if the patient has only been on a standard package Mediterranean holiday.

The commonest causes of a gastroenterinal infection in a patient recently returned from abroad are surprisingly almost the same as the indigenous United Kingdom infections. Toxigenic *E. coli* are the most likely cause of traveller's diarrhoea. Rotaviruses in children and campylobacter in adults are still very common. Particularly in adults, however, the rarer causes become more frequent. Salmonella infections are still a close second to campylobacter but the very rare causes like amoebic dysentery are almost exclusively imported. The rarer varieties of shigella dysentery like *Shigella shiga* and *S. boydii*, which are generally more vicious than *S. sonnei* dysentery, are almost always imported. *S. flexneri* dysentery has become more common in the UK but many strains of *S. flexneri* are still commonly imported.

Chronic diarrhoea

The patient who has a chronic low grade diarrhoea is the one in whom the travel history is most likely to be missed. *Giardia lam-*

blia is often the cause and although it is very common in Britain may only be diagnosed as an imported infection because the faeces have been microscopically examined, looking for the larger, but much less common, amoebic cysts.

The cysts of *G. lamblia* are notoriously difficult to see in faeces (principally because of their size) and the easier ways of diagnosis are far more unpleasant for the patient (duodenal aspiration and possible jejunal biopsy). Often the most practical way of dealing with a low grade, chronic, mild diarrhoea is a therapeutic trial. The best way of treating *G. lamblia* infection is a single large dose (2 g) of metronidazole on an empty stomach first thing in the morning for 2–3 consecutive days. This dosage is very nauseous and more recently tinidazole (also 2 g, but only four tablets as opposed to five to ten) as a single dosage has been more acceptable to some patients. Alcohol should be avoided with both preparations.

Jaundice

A patient presenting with jaundice having recently returned from abroad should be treated in the same way as a United Kingdom resident (see Chapter 9). Hepatitis A is as common, or commoner, in most parts of the world where United Kingdom residents holiday (except North America and Scandinavia) than in Britain, but the possibility of other causes of jaundice – malaria, yellow fever and amoebic liver abscess (usually presents as PUO) should be borne in mind. Hepatitis B is much commoner in other parts of the world (notably south-east Asia – see Chapter 9) but remember the incubation period has a mean time of 100 days and therefore hepatitis B would present some 2–3 months after return unless the period overseas was much longer than 2–3 weeks. Leptospirosis is commoner in most countries than in Britain and, as in Britain, is very much an occupational disease but occasionally a recreational one – e.g. fishing, other freshwater sports and caving (the last imported case in the Regional Infectious Diseases Unit in Manchester being a doctor who had been caving in Borneo).

Other febrile illnesses

Although malaria and enteric fever are important life-threatening infections most patients will have 'ordinary' infections and some will even have non-infectious causes of their fever. Unfortunately, the commonest cause of non-infection-related pyrexia of unknown origin is malignancy, but the ubiquitous viral infection will still be the commonest. Perhaps because the patients are more likely to be investigated when they have returned from abroad, influenza is probably confirmed more often when acquired on the Costa del Sol than Cleethorpes.

Skin rashes

Skin problems often occur after foreign travel, not least because of exposure to more ultraviolet light which can cause 'flare-ups' of herpes simplex or even more exotic conditions such as systemic lupus erythematosis.

Insect bites with, or without, allergic reactions are more common and occasionally exotic infections such as cutaneous leishmaniasis can be acquired on a Mediterranean holiday as well as further afield. They are all, of course, extremely rare.

Neurological

Neurological problems are relatively rare but the toxic confusional state is an obvious presentation of many infections.

ADVICE ON FOREIGN TRAVEL

When a patient consults his/her doctor before travelling abroad it is usually for either immunizations or *a repeat prescription*.

The opportunity should be taken for some general hygienic advice. Most holidaymakers are ill when on holiday because of overindulgence (usually either too much alcohol or too much sunshine, occasionally both) and sound advice on moderation is timely. Sensible advice on *only* eating properly cooked food and *only* drinking 'safe' water is necessary. For travellers to developing countries, water purifying tablets and straws with bacterial filters are available, but these exotic precautions are unnecessary for most holidaymakers.

In addition, if the traveller is going by pressurized aircraft there are some additional rules[4]. In general, the traveller has to be completely recovered from any recent illness – 10 days after minor surgery and 21 days after major surgery are general guidelines. Current illnesses to be particularly wary of are otitis media and sinusitis and at least a week should have passed since air or carbon dioxide was introduced or present in body cavities (the commonest occurrence would probably be laparoscopy).

If the travellers are going on a watersports holiday, remind them that sub aqua activities should cease at least 48 hours before the return journey.

Not only 'where?' but 'how?' and 'why?' have obvious medical implications beyond friendly curiosity.

In general, pregnancy beyond 35 weeks on flights over 2–3 hours, and 36 weeks on all flights, is severely frowned upon (see almost any airline ticket).

IMMUNIZATION FOR FOREIGN TRAVEL

The main thing to remember is that local rules are made to protect the visited not the visitors. Although when in doubt it can be useful to ring the appropriate Embassy about what is necessary to enter, what is necessary often falls short of what is the best protection for the traveller.

Immunization certificates

There are only two international immunization certificates, those for cholera and yellow fever.

Yellow fever

Yellow fever vaccination (officially lasts 10 years) is only available from special centres and is necessary for travellers to northern

South America (including parts of Central America), and Africa south of the Sahara (figure 13.2).

Contraindications

As in live virus vaccine the usual contraindications are pregnancy and immunosuppression (see Chapter 2). Additional contraindications are allergy to eggs, neomycin or polymyxin. It is a very effective vaccination, thus the 10-year-valid certificate. Yellow fever immunization should *not* be given to children under 1 year old.

Cholera vaccine

Cholera vaccine is a killed whole bacterial preparation and is generally regarded as one of the least effective vaccines currently available. The international certificate lasts 6 months.

Primary course

The primary course is usually two s.c./i.m. doses, 4 or more weeks apart (first = 0.5 ml; second = 1.0 ml). This interval can be reduced if necessary, and less local reaction follows intradermal (i.d.) injection, but this i.d. route (0.2 ml) should be used for second dose and boosters only. Smaller doses can be given to children.

Cholera immunization should *not* be given to children under 1 year old.

The relative ineffectiveness of the cholera vaccine usually means it should only be given when it is a requirement of entry.

Typhoid vaccine (monovalent)

This is recommended to all travellers outside northern Europe, Canada, the United States, Australia and New Zealand. It is currently recommended by the Department of Health and Social Security for all Mediterranean holidaymakers and the typhoid outbreak on the Greek island of Kos produced a panic of urgent demand for typhoid vaccine. It was completely pointless immun-

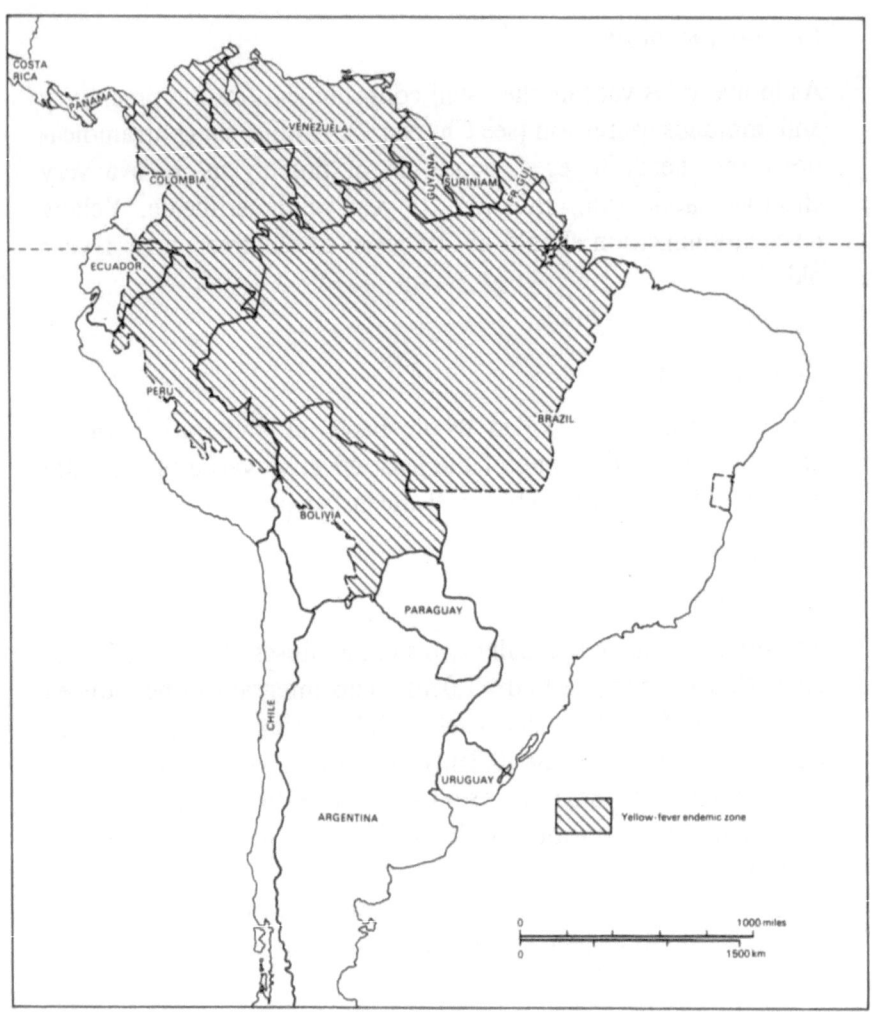

Figure 13.2   Yellow fever endemic zones in the Americas and Africa

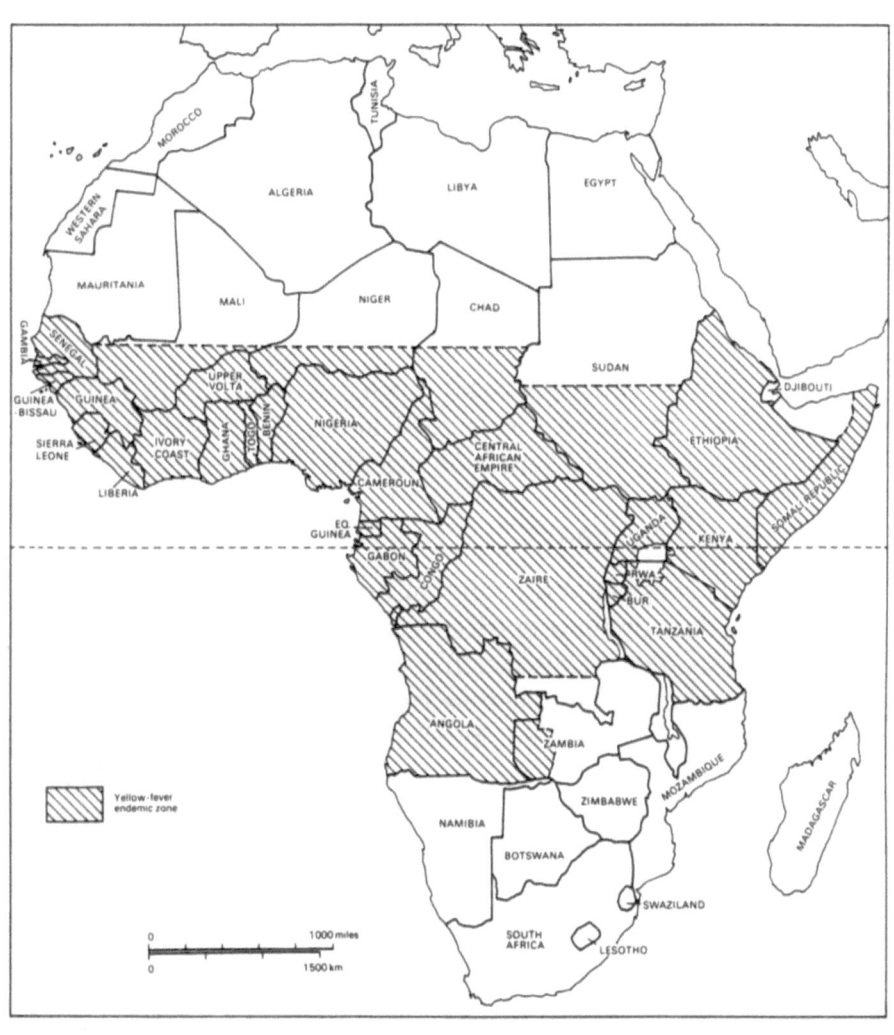

Yellow-fever
endemic zone

0 — 1000 miles
0 — 1500 km

izing package holidaymakers at the airport, particularly as *most* of them were going many thousands of miles away from the outbreak – the immunization was only just proving some protection for the return journey home. In general, the authors do not recommend immunization for ordinary Mediterranean holidaymakers unless they are travelling to the eastern Mediterranean (Turkey, Greece) or North Africa (Morocco or Tunisia). Those people going on low budget holidays (camping etc) have a greater need to be immunized:

initial dose: 0.5 ml s.c./i.m.
second dose: 0.1 ml intradermal

The intradermal route produces much less local reaction. The initial dose can be halved for children under 10 years and again children *under the age of 1 year* should *not* be immunized.

Immunization of children

If it is absolutely essential for children to visit, or live with, parent or parents in developing countries where extra immunizations are necessary, it should not distract from the fact that the most important immunizations are the *primary course triple* (tetanus, diphtheria and polio). In addition, measles vaccine can be given with some considerable benefit from 9 months of age onwards. BCG immunization is also strongly recommended for all who are tuberculin skin test negative.

Polio immunization

Polio immunization (see Chapter 2) is a live oral vaccine and can be given as a single booster to all adults up to 50 years of age; for those over 50, some authorities (M.M.W.R. supplement, 28.9.84) recommend inactivated polio vaccine (s.c./i.m.). The risk of vaccine-associated paralysis is greater with older recipients but is still incredibly rare (one case for 6.7 million doses).[5]

Oral polio vaccine contains a large number of antibiotics and the inactivated i.m. route should be used to anyone who is generally allergic to penicillin, streptomycin and kanamycin. Neomycin and polymyxin are present in both preparations.

Tetanus and diphtheria

Any adult attending for immunizations for foreign travel should be asked about tetanus and diphtheria and immunized accordingly. Remember adults should only be given diphtheria toxoid *after* Shick testing (positive requires immunization).

Hepatitis

Hepatitis B vaccine (see Chapter 9) can be used particularly for travellers to West Africa and south-east Asia but at the moment is only available to high risk groups such as health care workers. Medical student electives are a very good indication but few are taking the opportunity as yet.

Prophylaxis against hepatitis A when travelling to developing countries is indicated for those over 12 and under 50 years of age.

Remember that the protection is short lived (see Chapter 9).

Bitten abroad[6]

Occasionally a general practitioner may be consulted by a patient on return to the United Kingdom when they have been bitten whilst out of the country. Dogs and cats are usually the culprits and unfortunately the most important information is not usually available. Precise information about the animal is needed. If someone is bitten on the beach in Spain (which is technically rabies-free) the dog may have come from Germany or France as there are no import restrictions on animals. If the dog/cat is alive and well 3 weeks later, it did not have rabies. In the case of smaller animals, e.g. squirrels or skunks, the same is unfortunately not true, as they can carry the virus in their saliva and remain well.

The current rabies vaccine is very safe, very effective and much less painful than previous preparations. It is made in human tissue culture (not duck embryo or rabbit brain) which accounts for most of its better properties. It is given i.m. or deep s.c. Reactions are very rare but five or six injections are necessary. Unfortunately, the vaccine is not available on the NHS when taken prophylactically. Post-exposure boosters are recommended even for those previously immunized. Other animals than those named above, particularly monkeys, can cause problems, but often other infections such as herpes simplex (simian) are more important than rabies. Specialist advice should be sought at the first consultation.

REFERENCES

1. Reid, D., Dewar, R.D., Fallon, R.J., Cossar, J. H. and Crist, N. R. (1980). Infection and travel. *J. Infect.*, **2**, 365-70
2. C.D.R. 84/30. 27 July, 1984
3. Bruce-Chwatt, L. J. (1983). Malaria and pregnancy. *Br. Med. J.*, **286**, 1457-8
4. Walker, E. and Williams, G. (1983) *Br. Med. J.*, **286**, 865
5. WHO Consultative Group (1982). *Bull. WHO*, **60** (No. 2)
6. Ministry of Agriculture, Fisheries and Food and the Central Office of Information (1984)

14

Good Standards

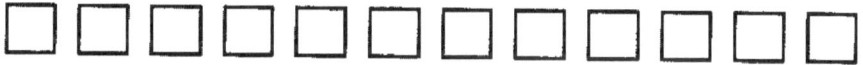

All of us are anxious to provide high quality care for our patients and most of us are interested in developing ideas about whether or not we are doing it. This chapter seeks to improve standards of care in the management of patients with infection in general practice.

WHAT DOES AUDIT MEAN?

There is a tendency to confuse the words 'research' and 'audit'. This is a pity because, although many of us are put off by the thought of a research project, audit exercises ought to be carried out by all of us from time to time if we are concerned to find out about what we do as opposed to what we think we do – more of this later. Both research and audit have to do with asking questions, but in a different sort of way.

Audit is asking questions about whether or not our care matches the standards which *we* have decided we should follow. It is important that the standards we choose are our own rather than somebody else's and that they represent the basic level below which we would not wish to fall.

Research also asks questions but these are designed to lead to the production of new standards. Esssentially, research asks 'What are the standards of care that the profession should provide?' and audit asks 'Are we doing it?'

Research may require special skills and expertise depending on the nature of the questions. It certainly requires a particular sort of mind. Audit, on the other hand, need not involve special skills and should be within the capabilities of all of us.

WHAT CAN WE AUDIT?

In 1966 Donabedian clarified our thinking about audit when he pointed out that our professional work, all of it, can be considered under three headings – structures, process and outcome[1].

Structure

This refers to elements such as the doctor/patient ratio in society or in a practice, the membership and size of the primary health care team, the availability of diagnostic facilities such as dip slides, swabs, otoscopes, examination rooms.

Process

This relates to the way in which diagnoses are made and patients managed. It may relate, for example, to the number of times a child with recurrent urinary infection has a specimen checked for bacteriuria, and the quality of the investigation. It could relate to the diagnostic criteria selected and employed for acute otitis media, or the management plans adopted for acute gastroenteritis in infants or upper respiratory infection in adults.

Outcome

At the end of the day, success or failure is best judged in terms of outcome for the patient. This is, however, a very difficult exercise. At what stage in the natural history of a disease should the outcome be measured and by what criteria? Are disease outcomes all that matter? What about intermediate outcomes such as the outcome of the consultation? It is clearly unrealistic, for example, to expect the general practitioner to prevent renal scarring in all children at risk in his practice. On the other hand it is realistic to ask the general practitioner to avoid an ampicillin rash in all patients with glandular fever by making the simple decision not to prescribe the drug for sore throats and by enabling the patient to see the sense in this. The difficulty is agreeing the standards.

TYPES OF MEDICAL AUDIT

Two types of medical audit are described – group audit and self-audit.

Group audit

This may concern itself with structure, process or outcome and may take the form of a peer group audit with or without an expert external resource. Normally a group of interested general practitioners (say up to 12?) come together to evaluate problem-solving and clinical management. For example, how should we best care for patients with 'cystitis' in general practice? There are many ways of leading into the discussion, including the presentation of a random case or a problem case by one of the group members, the prior circulation of a paper, a 10-minute talk by a group member or an invited expert, an audio tape or videotape of a consultation involving the topic, or an attempt to produce a management flow chart (algorithm) such as for frequency and dysuria syndrome.

Such groups, when working well, can be a most effective method of medical audit and continuing education for any clinician – certainly far superior to the traditional postprandial Section 63 lectures which may only transfer a few items to improve our store of factual knowledge. They can be a powerhouse for the generation of new ideas. There are a few hazards, however. First of all, the group must be prepared to work. Secondly, group leaders must ensure that discussion does not degenerate into a levelling down to the lowest common denominator. One well-known teacher of general practice used to employ a technique in which he would ask a group of half a dozen experienced general practitioners to name the drug they would use if a young married woman presented with acute frequency and dysuria. He would

221

expect and get half a dozen different answers. He would conclude from this that there was no right answer as six experienced doctors behaved differently. An expert resource would point out that a correct choice should be based on safety, effectiveness and cost, which quickly limits the choice available.

Critical appraisal of cases may involve such questions as the following.

(1) Is the problem resolved in the shortest possible time?
(2) Have the number of problem-solving steps been reduced to the minimum?
(3) Has the simplest technology been employed?
(4) Does the clinical management plan cause minimum harm?
(5) Has the best use been made of health care personnel?
(6) Have self-care and family care been fully mobilized?

Self-audit

Any doctor can evaluate his conduct of a consultation by asking basic questions such as the following.

(1) Have I helped this patient?
(2) Could I have prevented a recurrence of this or associated problems?
(3) Have I acted with maximum economy and efficiency?
(4) Has anything important been omitted?
(5) Should I have referred this patient or enlisted the help of another agency?
(6) Am I the best doctor for this situation?

AUDIT IN PRACTICE

Some months ago one of the authors (DB) was aked to write an article on audit on otitis media for a well-known monthly medical journal. The first thing to do, he decided, was to agree some standards relating to structure, process and outcome. A simple matter, he thought. Partners were called together. We agreed

that we should have otoscopes available and with working bat-
teries! We agreed (just about) that both ears should be examined.
We agreed that children with earache should be seen quickly if
telephone advice about analgesia did not work, and at the next
available surgery if it did. We could not agree on the otoscopic
diagnostic criteria for otitis media or on whether antibiotics
should be prescribed and in what circumstances. We then turned
to what we regarded as minimal information to be recorded in the
notes after a consultation for otitis media. Did the side have to be
specified and recorded or the appearance of the drum? We did not
think so. The only essential information, we thought, was the
diagnosis and the drug treatment. This limited our audit exercise
considerably, as you can imagine.

I then remembered that I had written an article on otitis media
for *Update* in the past in which I had made statements about the
care I thought should be provided[2]. Essentially, I stated that I
gave analgesics and 'advice' to children with earache and pink
drums and antibiotics to children with earache and bulging red
drums. No drops or decongestants were prescribed. I said that
patients were followed up in 7–10 days for assessment (drum resolution and deafness). I said that further investigation and ENT
investigation were rare.

Table 14.1 presents data relating to an internal enquiry into

Table 14.1   An audit exercise for otitis media in general practice

1. 128 children were seen in the practice over a 12-month period

2. 34 were followed-up or came back

3. *Treatment*	*Patients (n)*
Amoxycillin	68
Ampicillin	9
Co-trimoxazole	9
Penicillin V	13
Erythromycin	9
Not recorded	20
4. Referral audiology	9
5. Referral ENT surgeon	6

whether or not the practice adhered to the standards I had (perhaps somewhat pompously) laid down! It was rather embarrassing to find out that if any children did not receive antibiotics they had to be found in a group of 20 children whose treatment was not recorded! Why is there this paranoia factor? Why did I think that I followed-up most children with otitis media? Is it really necessary anyway? Perhaps the population with glue ear is only obliquely related to the population with otitis media and there is little point in routine follow-up for the latter group.

ANTIBIOTICS IN ABUNDANCE? – AN ENQUIRY INTO ANTIBIOTIC PRESCRIBING IN ONE PRACTICE

During January, 1982, we saw more upper respiratory tract infection than we have ever seen in the 4 years we had been producing workload statistics. It was also the month when we decided that we would look at the pattern of antibiotic prescribing in our practice.

The data

Table 14.2 shows the total number of prescriptions for antibiotics issued during the study period (January 1982) and the disease categories into which the patients fell. By far the majority of

Table 14.2 Patients in certain disease categories and total number of prescriptions for antibiotics given in the practice within that category during January 1982

Disease	Patients (n)	Prescriptions (n)
Respiratory diseases	468	192
Skin diseases	71	45
Ear infections		35
Genito-urinary diseases	47	22
Infectious and parasitic diseases	56	14
Total	642	308

patients (468) had upper respiratory tract infections and 41% of all patients with respiratory infection were treated with an antibiotic. The number of patients with skin diseases totalled 71, and 63% of all patients with skin diseases were treated with an antibiotic. Of 47 patients with genito-urinary disease, 45% were treated with an antibiotic, as were 23% of 56 patients with infectious and parasitic disease.

Table 14.3 presents the age/sex breakdown of patients receiving

Table 14.3 Age/sex breakdown (%) of 308 practice patients receiving antibiotics during January 1982

Age group (y)	M	F	Total
0–4	22	17	39
5–14	21	22	43
15–29	25	37	62
30–44	12	29	41
45–64	20	37	57
65+	28	38	66
Total	128	180	308

antibiotics during January 1982. When comparisons are made with the age/sex distribution of the practice, it is clear that the very young and the very old are particularly well represented among the patients who received an antibiotic.

Table 14.4 lists the antibiotics prescribed. Amoxycillin (Amoxil), oxytetracycline (Terramycin), co-trimoxazole (Septrin) and penicillin V are clearly most favoured, with erythromycin (Erythrocin) a popular runner-up.

The lessons

The introduction of antibiotics nearly 50 years ago has not had much impact on the common infectious diseases. They are ineffective against most infections we encounter, and even vulnerable organisms develop resistance. Diseases change over the years and social and environmental factors have played a more prominent

Table 14.4   Antibiotics prescribed in the practice during January 1982

Antibiotic	Times prescribed (n)
Oxytetracycline (Terramycin)	60
Amoxycillin (Amoxil)	60
Co-trimoxazole (Septrin)	51
Penicillin V	45
Erythromycin (Erythrocin)	31
Ampicillin (Penbritin)	15
Metronidazole (Flagyl)	7
Flucloxacillin (Floxapen)	12
Others	17
Total	298

part than chemotherapy in the decline of many infections. Even before chemotherapy, the great majority of infections were resolved perfectly satisfactorily by natural body defence mechanisms. Our practice figures indicate the extent to which an ordinary practice has come to depend on antibiotics.

It was rather startling to discover that 63% of all patients with skin disease were treated with antibiotics, until we looked at individual prescriptions and discovered that most of these patients did not have eczema or psoriasis but boils, furuncles, cellulitis and paronychias, not to mention those with acne. We were relieved to note that only 41% of patients with respiratory disease were treated with antibiotics; this does show an attempt to be selective, as does the observation that more antibiotics were given to the very young and the very old. Two studies in north-east Scotland found that antibiotics were prescribed for just over half the new consultations for respiratory illness[3, 4].

We were also rather pleased to note that we were choosing simple antibiotics, but we are beginning to ask ourselves why we prescribe so much amoxycillin at twice the cost of ampicillin, and whether all our oxytetracycline prescriptions are appropriate? We are also relieved to discover that no prescription for an acute problem was issued without a direct consultation. However, four repeat scripts for oxytetracycline were given to patients with acne.

Moss and her colleagues[5] have reported a survey of antibiotic prescribing in a district general hospital. Twenty-eight per cent of all inpatients received antibiotics and, as in our practice, there was a greater tendency for older patients to receive them. Ampicillin (or amoxycillin) accounted for over 40% of the prescriptions and was the most popular choice. We were interested to discover that most patients in Moss's study were treated without bacteriological evidence of the infecting agent and that in 50% of cases prescribers were unable to specify the pathogens against which treatment was intended. We felt that we would do better in terms of identifying the expected pathogens but we would doubt the value of bacteriological investigation for routine infections in general practice, except perhaps in some patients (especially children) with urinary infections.

Strictly speaking, this 'enquiry' was not an audit exercise as we had agreed no standards beforehand against which we could measure our prescribing behaviour as a practice. We merely 'reacted' to the data produced. All the evidence suggests, however, that we should be much more selective with our scripts for antibiotics. Controlled trials have shown no difference in the outcome of acute otitis media in children treated with antibiotics or placebos[6]. The course of tonsillitis may be shortened by one day with the use of penicillin. Most acute urinary tract infections will cure themselves. Stott, studying upper respiratory infections, showed that there was no difference in outcome, in terms of complications or reattendance rate, in children consulting general practitioners who prescribed antibiotics frequently and those who prescribed them hardly at all[7].

Perhaps we should make attempts to evaluate our own prescribing patterns. Such exercises could well be attempted and discussed in practices or continuing education groups. Why do we prescribe antibiotics for 5-7 days? Patients with streptococcal throat infections should receive 14 days treatment to prevent a recurrence and perhaps other throat infections don't need penicillin at all? Do frequent prescribers teach their patients that antibiotics are needed for common family illnesses and that a visit to a doctor is therefore necessary? Why are we so ready to change our prescribing habits after visits by drug firm representatives who enthuse about their new 'Wondercillin'?

COMMON-SENSE PRESCRIBING

Having said all this, however, the author is reminded of an incident in which he declined to prescribe penicillin when a young man presented with a sore throat and no physical signs. The patient was a well-known television entertainer and was very anxious about his next performance. The doctor, however, was anxious about the man's high-pressure lifestyle and wondered whether he was drinking too much. The decision not to give penicillin ruined the consultation and an opportunity to build up a continuing relationship was destroyed. Although the entertainer is still a patient, he rarely consults us, preferring to have frequent health checks at a local BUPA centre. We receive pages of normal laboratory investigations, but we suspect that the heavy drinking and smoking could continue and that the underlying health anxieties and hazards which lead to the BUPA checks are being neglected. An opportunity for anticipatory care has been lost (possibly for ever) for the sake of a few penicillin tablets. The author is left with an uncomfortable feeling and the growing certainty that he made a mistake, and that among the indications for antibiotic therapy in general practice must be included a few that are 'social' or 'psychological'. Time to educate about penicillin when the relationship exists. Perhaps part of the appeal of general practice is that there are few certainties, and that prescribing must be based on common sense as well as scientific method.

REFERENCES

1. Donabedian, A. (1966). Evaluating the quality of medical care. *Milbank Mem. Fund Q.*, **44,** 166-206
2. Brooks, D. (1983). Otitis media. *Update*, 1 June
3. Howie, J.G.R., Richardson, I.M., Gill, G. and Curno, D. (1971). Respiratory illness and antibiotic use in general practice. *J. R. Coll. Gen. Practit.*, **21,** 657-63
4. Howie, J.G.R. (1973). A new look at respiratory illness in general practice. *J. R. Coll. Gen. Practit.*, **23,** 895-904
5. Moss, F., McSwiggan, D.A., McNicol, M.W. and Miller, D.L. (1981). Survey of antibiotic prescribing in a district general hospital. Pattern of use. *Lancet*, **3,** 349-51
6. Van Buchem, F.L., Donk, J.H.M. and Vant Hoff, M.A. (1981).

Therapy of acute otitis media: Myringotomy antibiotics or neither. A double blind study in children. *Lancet*, **2,** 883–7

7. Stott, N.C.H. (1979). Management and outcome of winter upper respiratory tract infections in children aged 0–9. *Br. Med. J.*, **1,** 29–31

Index